HEALING
CHRONIC BACK PAIN

7 STEPS TO PERFECT POSTURE

Order Your Personal Copy From

OrthoWellness Publications

www.HealingChronicBackPain.com

****SECURE Internet Book Orders****

HEALING
CHRONIC BACK PAIN

7 STEPS TO PERFECT POSTURE

Mark Frobb M.D.

OrthoWellness Publications

ISBN 1-4196-2482-2
LCCN 2006901406

To Order Additional Copies
Contact
OrthoWellness Publications
1661-128 St.
Surrey, British Columbia
Canada V4A 3V2
604-531-0444

Library of Congress Cataloguing-in-Publication Data
Library of Congress Control Number: 2006901406
Publisher: BookSurge, LLC
North Charleston, South Carolina

Healing Chronic Back Pain:
7 Steps to Perfect Posture
Mark Frobb MD

(1) HEALTH & FITNESS / General   (2) HEALTH & FITNESS / Exercise
(3) HEALTH & FITNESS / Healing   (4) MEDICAL / General
(5) SELF-HELP / General

1. Chronic back pain 2. Posture Exercises 3. Spinal Therapy
4. Pain Management 5. Chronic Pain Treatment

Artwork and cover design by Donna Mendes

*… to those that suffer and
the therapists charged with their care*

ACKNOWLEDGMENTS

Every practicing physician is a product of the mentors who have graciously expended energy in sharing their knowledge and experience in the healing arts, and I have been fortunate to count many throughout my 30-year medical career. This personal foundation of medical knowledge not surprisingly can cover a vast landscape of contributing teachers, in my case, from experiences with my father who practiced for 40 years as a country practitioner in Northern Canada, to my association with Dr. Christiaan Barnard, the world's first heart transplant surgeon from South Africa.

The treatment management of Chronic Back Pain is as much of an art as it is a science. With the complexity of the etiology leading to its onset, and the mix of myofascial and neuropathic pain presentations, it is not unreasonable that the best practitioners are those that have the widest variety of treatment approaches in their therapeutic armamentarium.

As one of my mentors once put it; "If the only tool you have in your bag is a hammer, everything will start to look like a nail."

In pursuit of this syllabus of continuing education, I have had had the privilege of training in a renaissance era of manual medicine with opportunities of participation in hands-on treatment workshops with the giants of Osteopathic manual therapy, including Drs. Janet Travell, John Mennell, Philip Greenman and John Bordillion, as well as the renowned physiotherapist from Australia, Robin McKenzie.

The adjunctive study of Traditional Chinese Medicine, with an entirely new set of mentors including Drs. Steven Aung, Joseph Wong, Sona Tahan and Linda Rapson along with over a decade of study in Taijiquan, the accompanying exercise companion to Traditional Chinese Medicine, has added an entirely new dimension and paradigm shift to my understanding and treatment of Chronic Back Pain.

The footnotes, articles and references that are accumulated during the writing of a book eventually fill multiple filing cabinet drawers and it is difficult to credit all the great contributors to medical science as the knowledge base evolves from decade to decade in the understanding of complex medical problems.

In the writing of this particular book however, I would like to acknowledge reference to the excellent anthology prepared by David Yosifon and Peter N. Stearns on the cultural history of posture. Although these historical facts are cross-referenced extensively in public archives, it is access to this type of documented research that assists authors in covering vast tracts of time quickly, saving innumerable research hours. It is to these authors and others who have tirelessly researched and presented the multitude of tidbits of facts that comprise the body of knowledge on a subject that I wish to express my thanks. It is only because of these efforts that the vanguard practitioners of today can assimilate and create new models of therapy in treatment of complex medical problems such as Chronic Back Pain.

In creating the title of the book, the word "healing" is used advisedly. The 16th-century French surgeon, Ambroise Pare wrote "I dressed the wound, it was God who healed it." 500 years later, this succinct observation is no less true. A therapist's role in the treatment of chronic back pain is a mere smoothing of the obstructions along the path to recovery. The healing remains within the realm of the body itself.

And lastly in the preparation of this book, I would like to graciously thank my editor, Donna Grant who spent so many hours interspersed within her exceptionally busy life honing my words to achieve needed clarity and my incredibly talented artist wife, Donna Mendes for her drawings which "instilled life into the words", conveying the kinesthetic images to the reader.

CONTENTS

PART II:
THE 7 PROMISES OF PERFECT POSTURE

PART III:
THE 7 SECRETS OF PERFECT POSTURE

PART IV:
THE SEVEN STEPS TO PERFECT POSTURE

Reading Notes:

PART I

UNRAVELLING THE MYSTERY OF CHRONIC BACK PAIN

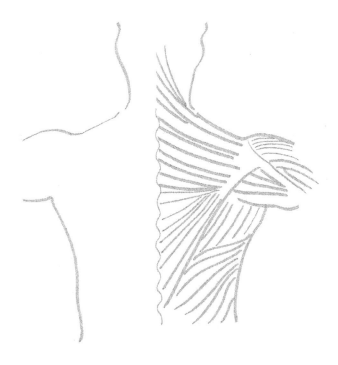

Using Personal Empowerment in the Treatment of Chronic Back Pain

1

O nly 3% of all causes of back pain can be attributed to a significant pathological process, even when drawing upon the most advanced medical investigative tools available today. Within this very small group are included the pathological diagnoses of tumors, fractures, infections, spinal cord and nerve root pressure syndromes, abdominal or pelvic organ diseases, rheumatoid and other autoimmune arthritic disorders, and various other systemic diseases, which may produce back pain.

The overwhelming 97% of back pain sufferers remaining have what is widely discussed in the medical literature as "non-specific back pain". Back pain specialists accept the term "non-specific back pain" as a clinical diagnosis, representing a clinical syndrome whose foundation probably stems from a multidimensional musculoskeletal health problem.

The most common feature in examination of patients presenting with "chronic, non-specific back pain syndrome", is an aberration from normal postural alignment. This association is so common that one might almost be tempted to call chronic, *non-specific* back pain, chronic, *postural* back pain.

Some critics might regard this statement as presumptuous if the attempt is to imply that the postural changes were causative and, therefore, predated the back pain. A different argument might presuppose that the observed postural changes were a result of deliberate changes to postural alignment, made by the afflicted patient, in a naturally adopted pain management strategy used to find the most comfortable position to improve a pre-existing back pain syndrome.

Chronic back pain is one of the top 5 reasons for doctor visits in North America

This may very well be true in the initial stages, but persistence of this altered dysfunctional postural alignment, as we will see, will lead to loss of core strength and postural balance, which produces the end result of chronic back pain in any case, making a moot point of the entire argumentative exercise.

With each passing decade since the 1950s, the incidence of chronic back pain syndrome has become increasingly more endemic in industrialized countries and is now ranked within the top five most common reasons for visits to physicians' offices in North America. When one thinks of all the technologically advanced investigative and treatment costs related to heart disease, cancer and the many chronic diseases like diabetes, it comes as a shock to find that the total medical dollars spent on investigation and treatment of the lowly chronic back pain syndrome ranks in the top six of health care costs. When considering the resultant absenteeism and extra secondary costs to trade and industry, this economic burden extends far beyond the direct medical costs.

The Financial and Personal Cost of Chronic Back Pain

Aside from the financial burden, there are immeasurable personal costs associated with chronic back pain as individuals attempt to cope with their disability, struggling through the activities of daily life in which many find their enjoyment markedly compromised. Because of its epidemic proportions, significant injurious impact

4

on life and associated expense, any solution that will impact upon this trend and reduce disability associated with chronic back pain will have a tremendous potential for improving population health standards and freeing up valuable health resources.

As the many suffering individuals pursue their personal search for this Holy Grail, many billions of dollars are spent annually as back pain sufferers trek from therapist to therapist, looking for the solution to their suffering. Rarely is a solution predictably found with any given modality of therapy, with treatment response significantly marked by idiosyncrasy, a medical term suggesting that what works for one person may not necessarily work for the next. In fact, what worked the first time for an individual may not necessarily work the next.

The Revolving Door of Chronic Back Pain Treatment

Many chronic back pain patients will go through this revolving door of treatment scores of times as they live through the cycle of exacerbation and remission marking the natural history of chronic postural back pain. Desperate but hopeful as they hear stories of success from friends and acquaintances who swear by their current therapist, they try yet another treatment modality in their search for the magic bullet that will make the problem go away.

Even if we do find someone who can help us out of our current "bad stretch" of back pain, we can unnervingly find ourselves tied to a particular therapist as we struggle to maintain the tenuous balance in this

> Billions of dollars are spent annually as back pain sufferers search for the Holy Grail of pain relief

unending battle with the chronic back pain syndrome. With this loss of empowerment, it is easy to attach uneasy power to this person whom we think holds the key to making us feel better, worrying about holiday scheduling (both theirs and ours), always fearful that something will go wrong.

Does Posture Play a Role in Chronic Back Pain?

Everyone has heard that one of the keys to improving back pain is correction of posture. Most of us even have a vague idea of what good posture is. We are reminded of our parents' exhortations to straighten up and walk tall. Perhaps even some of us are aware of privileged childhood classmates who were shipped off to elite finishing schools where the final touches in body carriage, manners and other societal niceties were entrenched and embodied.

Most probably, however, we took these exhortations with a grain of salt, carried on in our own way and thought little of it again. Perhaps it is time to revisit this issue of posture. All the medical evidence suggests that ergonomically erect posture plays a key role in the treatment of chronic back pain. In fact, regardless of what other therapeutic modalities we may bring to bear in treatment of chronic back pain, unless effort is made to correct the faulty posture, little lasting progress will be made in alleviation of this common, disabling pain syndrome.

The Cultural History of Posture

2

From a woman's claim of respectability to a man's ascendance in military rank, posture has played a key historical role in depicting our place in society.

Posture in Ancient History

An artistic appreciation of youthful posture, as represented in Greco-Roman sculpture and ancient Egyptian and Asian art, presented the only tangible reference to posture prior to the mid-1700s. Little mention of it ever appeared in the medical writings of the day or any other literature, for that matter.

Good posture, however, has always been linked with a proper military bearing. Poor or languid postures were commonly associated with a lack of discipline and even a dereliction of duty in military ranks. Accordingly, the stance of "at attention" has always denoted alertness and a special sensory awareness of immediate surroundings. A physically demonstrable respect for ranking officials and officers is also commonly conveyed through posture. This military bearing crosses cultural boundaries and appears in almost all societies, wherever there are clear-cut divisions of rank.

In the Eastern philosophies of martial arts, good posture was identified as a necessary fundamental and preparatory stance to achieve success in combat. The ancient martial arts treatises that have survived from antiquity have dealt carefully and clearly with the teaching of perfect posture to the acolytes of the warrior classes. Because many of these early martial arts masters shared traditional roles as spiritual teachers, it was not unreasonable that the same tenements of proper posture would be adopted into meditative poses—practices that have survived into the present day.

Posture in the 1700s and the Victorian Age

In the secular organization of society prior to the mid-1700s, little attention was paid to proper posture. Leisurely slouching and a relaxed decorum generally marked the social settings depicted in art. Attentiveness to posture began to change, however, as cultural authorities of the day—Lord Chesterfield being one of them—began writing extensively on social interaction and manners, making specific reference to posture and "body carriage". For the next 150 years, considerable attention would be addressed to postural presentation, and its cultural effects would be widely seen in architecture and design, art, dance and general social interaction.

Published caricatures presented failures of society in hunched and slouched postures

The emphasis on formality and bodily dignity would be seen as a means to distinguish oneself from those who displayed an undisciplined lifestyle. Published caricatures would present failures of society in hunched and slouched postures, suggesting poor posture as a key contributor to a lack of success and perhaps even a cause of moral degradation.

The standard of the day would be the adoption of a proper posture, constituting a demonstration of a good and moral character. It implied a disciplined lifestyle, the ability to overcome physical weakness as well as the ability to control unbridled human desire. In some circles, these rules may have been so unfairly enforced that a woman's claim to respectability could be easily questioned if her posture suggested a careless or lounging attitude without watchful attention to proper body carriage.

The introduction of Darwinism in the early 19th-century contributed further to this popular support of erect posture, with educational charts demonstrating the continuum of ape to man, carefully commemorating increasingly better posture in each of the developmental stages. This resulted in an increased fervor for posture, with a cultural emphasis on proper posture both in child-rearing and school settings.

> A rapid change in postural standards was viewed as "the beginning of the end"

Comfort was not in the lexicon of posture vocabulary, and seating arrangements were almost always deliberately designed with back-less benches. Sitting-room furniture generally encouraged careful posture, with wooden and stiff-backed chairs adorned with light upholstery more for fashion than comfort. Even the rocking chair drew frowns from the "posture police" because of its relaxed qualities, which encouraged more of a lounging position. Its proper position in the hierarchy of seating would find it quickly relegated to the nursery and bedroom, where it was reserved for the exclusive use of nursing mothers or the aged and invalid.

These postural norms were also reflected in clothing styles, particularly in women, where elaborate undergarments—especially corsets—reflected constraint and formality. In men, the styles promoting a proper posture were equally mirrored with stiffly tailored formal coats and vests that insured upright postures both standing and sitting.

The Dawn of Modernism in Posture and the Declining Reign of Emily Post

With the beginning of the 20th century, some "chinks in the armor" of the postural proponents would begin to become evident—especially in North America where, culturally and economically, the New World was taking its place as an up-and-coming leader. The growing resistance to formally constrained posture in social

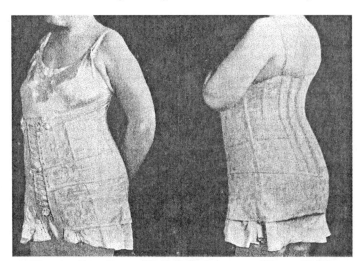

Illustration from Mail Catalogue--- Circa 1900

settings would become so widespread that, within a short decade, home furnishing factories (as illustrated in the advertisements of the American Sears catalog) were now promoting the sale of a wide selection of richly stuffed parlor seats. This rapid change in postural standards was viewed with alarm by many of the cultural gurus, as the beginning of the end. This arrogant challenge to the elegant propriety of the Victorian era even resulted in changes in architectural language, with "parlors" becoming "living rooms".

These changes dictated that the newly relaxed physical environment could no longer control the posture of the guests. The goal of the new socialite hostess would be to provide an easy, pleasant atmosphere, rather than the encouragement of stiff and formal restraints as imposed by the old-fashioned parlor.

The loss of corseting and other constraints standard in women's clothing, and the introduction of more freedom of movement in men's suits, allowed for greater relaxation of posture and quickly reflected in fashion, the new cultural transformations.

These revolutionary trends were embraced not only in North America, but Europe as well, with a growing acceptance of relaxation in social settings. Reclining—if not sprawling—could be seen in the many parks that were constructed at the beginning of the 20th century. With the introduction of the radio, the evening listening sessions promoted informal settings with bodies plopped in deeply upholstered chairs and sofas, arms and legs draped over chair arms and end tables, or simply spread out on the floor amongst cushions.

There would be fundamental changes in popular dance styles, with rigid, elegant waltzes transplanted from Europe replaced by new dances including the Cakewalk, Charleston and Jitterbug, especially influenced by African-American, Caribbean and other regional dance genres. Even classical ballet performances would lose some of the rigid postures and stiffness while continuing to preserve the grace and bodily control inherent in the art.

These changes were not universally accepted, with many established icons opposing the dissolution of Victorian standards. Emily Post, in response to these radical changes, published a series of etiquette manuals beginning in the 1920s. Seating at the table was a particular focus of proper posture and, like most of her Victorian predecessors, Emily Post wanted no compromise in erect posture. She was particularly firm in the instruction of children, insisting that they "be prevented from developing a careless attitude in seating that all too readily can generate into flopping this way and that."

With the postural changes rapidly overcoming society, Bancroft, Post and other contemporaries would form the American Posture League in 1914, in an attempt to preserve the norms of the Victorian standards. Much like the "Just Say No!" anti-drug campaigns of the 1990s, the campaign was very simple. Good posture, it was taught, reflected good living habits and bad posture reflected a mark of poor personal values.

The American Posture League, directed by leading orthopedic physicians of the day, physical education specialists and efficiency engineers, would enjoy a 30-year lifespan, surviving into the 1950s, yielding considerable influence and contributing widely to education. Amongst its activities, the League would contribute significantly to the research, development and publishing of educational literature designed to teach Americans the importance of postural self-discipline. Scientists committed to the ergonomics of posture would even contribute to the ergonomic design of public seating, designs that survive into modern-day architecture.

The return of war in the 1940s resulted in a resurgence of interest in posture, as militarism encouraged erect posture and school children were re-infected with the desire to mimic the heroes of the day. This was especially true when children were told that the posture training they were practicing every day, was derived from the very same programs instituted in the Officer and Cadet Armed Forces training camps. Posters in classrooms across America exhorted students to hold themselves high and proud and help win the war against tyranny.

During this period of revival, parents were expected to reinforce the evils of posture slumps in their children. Even pediatricians were caught up in this renaissance of posture training and, with the economic introduction of household cameras, photographs were introduced into medical records, serially recording postural changes of their patients from toddlers to school-age children and into early adulthood. This practice would even be adopted in university and colleges where both male and female entrants would be serially photographed from their freshman year onward, charting any changes that might suggest deterioration in posture and, thus, the need for intervention therapy.

> Posture programs became a regular part of institutional education, from kindergarten to higher learning

The Posture Clinic was soon to follow, where a child might be referred for correction of what was observed to be a change from the normally accepted postural charts, by a school official or physician. These postural charts were universally displayed in physicians' offices, schools and other institutions and organizations where children were grouped together.

Posture programs were a regular part of the institutional educational curriculum from kindergarten into higher learning. The Department of Physical Education issued regular "posture bulletins" to institutions within their jurisdiction, and grading on children's report cards specifically commented on postural attainment.

Posture and the Age of Dr. Spock

In the early 1950s, Dr. Benjamin Spock's classic work on children changed generally accepted attitudes in parenting. It would be suggested that overzealous parental nagging constituted a counterproductive child-rearing philosophy. The new psychological teaching would advise that posture problems might be the manifestation rather than the cause of developmental problems, perhaps harboring other elements or difficulties, including psychological problems and lack of self-confidence. Proponents of the new psychological theories suggested poor posture in itself could occur as a result of too much criticism at home or school, or be a reflection of difficulties with achievement or an unsatisfactory social life. The new child-rearing manuals and established experts now recommended that parents should restrict themselves in remarking on a child's posture. Poor posture would no longer be a matter for discipline of any sort; now the influence would be on making children proud of their bodies. Posture, good or bad, did not enter into this discussion one way or another.

Past theories that a healthy child would perform their activities more successfully if they resembled an alert soldier, became derided as an aesthetic ideal, which held no basis in fact, and was quickly labeled as a yesteryear cultism. No longer was posture considered a reflection of character or personal adjustment.

> Postural aids have rapidly developed into a multi-billion-dollar industry

Even within medical circles, there was a tendency to move away from the thought that posture could affect function of internal organs or cause changes in spinal alignment resulting in back pain. On the other hand, this was the same medical cohort that was suggesting that cigarette smoking was an excellent way to control appetite and nervousness. As one might expect, many of these extremist views reflected the inevitable swinging of the pendulum.

Even the new gurus of etiquette, like Amy Vanderbilt, while admiring wistfully the yesteryears of Victorian posture, were forced to admit the inevitable: "Today, with fewer and fewer uncompromising chairs being manufactured, we are more or less forced to lounge as we sit." Judith Martin's *Miss Manners*, published in the early 1980s, however, applauded the changing culture and humorously noted the fact that, for the first time in a longtime, a less formal posture could no longer be punishable by hanging.

More recently, we find an increasing supply of "postural aids" being marketed for the treatment of back and neck pain—from lumbar supported seating to mattresses with "deep down firmness for luxuriously relaxing support" to contoured neck supports and pillows. From humble beginnings this market quickly developed into a multi-billion-dollar industry, with consumers hungrily seeking easy solutions to the ever-increasing incidence of backache and neck pain.

The Renaissance of Posture Today

Not surprisingly, toward the end of the 20th century, we began to see a second renaissance in posture training. The broad recognition that core strength training and proper posture are the predominant treatment / prevention fundamentals for the vast majority of back and neck pain, provides the impetus behind this current posture renaissance. It also most certainly reinforces the fact that, of all the variety of treatments for back and neck maladies, without the strengthening of the core musculature and the correction of postural alignment, there remains little hope of correcting the cause of the common backache.

With the realization that normal postural alignment is the single most important factor in the prevention and maintenance of a healthy back, we have now come full circle in the evolution of our attitudes toward posture.

The Cultural History of Posture

Reading Notes:

The History of Surgical and Medical Intervention in Chronic Back Pain

3

The Mystique of Surgery

Treatments used in the intervention of back pain, both historically as well as in modern time, can be divided into two categories: surgical and non-surgical. The surgical interventions, although dramatic—especially from a historical perspective—represent a heroic approach in treatment for what were often life-threatening complications. Surprisingly, they play a small role in the treatment of backache today.

One of history's earliest documentations referring to surgical intervention in the treatment of back disorders was made by Galen, the original founding father of Greek medicine, who published a teaching text on spinal disorders in the 2nd century A.D. Other references in Western medicine have been noted in texts dating back to 700 to 900 A.D., and have been documented in Middle Eastern publications dating back to the time of ancient Arabia. Turkish surgeons in the 15th century also published several texts outlining surgical techniques for treatment of spinal disorders.

Recognizing that conventional anesthesia, as we know it today, would not be discovered until the late 19th-century, these original surgical techniques would not have been easy operations to carry out. Initially, the concept of surgical anesthesia was a mere dulling of the senses, consigned to the ingestion of large amounts of alcohol, the smoking or ingestion of hashish or opium, or simple concussion caused by placing a wooden bowl over the head of the unfortunate patient and clubbing him until consciousness was lost. Most often, however, the alert and struggling patient was forcibly restrained by surgical assistants through the course of the surgical procedure—or at least until the patient mercifully lost consciousness.

It would be in 18th-century London, with the widespread publication and documentation of surgical procedures and the formation of scientific societies, that the art of surgery would emerge with strength, developing standardizations in operative technique and management. Survival of the patient in these early hospital operating rooms, even under the hands of the most famous surgeons such as John Hunter, was not exemplary and probably dependent as much on the speed of the surgeon as his technical prowess.

It would not be until the discovery of ether as an effective surgical anesthetic at the end of the 19th century, that surgeons would have the leisure of operating on predictably unconscious patients over a period of hours, rather than the harried and rushed procedures on a struggling patient held down by surgical assistants, themselves doing their utmost to stay out of harm's way.

> Not until the end of the 19th century did surgeons have the luxury of operating on predictably unconscious patients

The swiftness and exacting sequence of the operation required the abject attention of the entire surgical team with little room for error. Given the flurry of activity, it was not surprising to find, on occasion, members of the surgical team inadvertently injured. As was duly recorded in one distinguished surgeon's journal, "the operation was marred by the unfortunate amputation of three fingers of my hapless assistant, who inattentively placed his hand in the path of my opening incision."

Those patients surviving the shock and rigors of the surgeon's knife would still face the very real perils of infection in the convalescent wards, where antiseptic standards were yet to be discovered and introduced. With little attention to cleanliness, the early era surgeons proudly wore their bloodstained aprons throughout the hospital as a recognizable uniform of their profession and a badge of honor. It would not be for the better part of a century and the discovery of the bacterium, that this practice would be observed as a significant lapse in infection control, responsible for widespread sepsis and subsequent mortality in post-surgical wards.

Understandably, it was the military campaigns of the day and the expertise of military surgeons that provided the setting for surgical training and progress in the management of major spinal trauma. Penetrating projectiles, severe lacerations and crush injuries would all be addressed as surgical emergencies with the hope of offering survival to the afflicted combatant.

The Introduction of Anesthesia

The beginning of the 20th century would herald a new era in the treatment of surgical management of spinal disorders. The capability of providing surgical anesthesia for long periods of time, coupled with the means of performing surgery under sterile technique, provided surgeons with a new and exciting theater in which to make significant advances in the offering of relief for many patients suffering from back pain.

Procedures were developed for removal of herniated discs pressing on spinal nerves, for correction of spinal canal stenosis (a compression causing constriction of the spinal cord and deteriorating neurological function), and for rectification of severe scoliosis by the implanting of steel rods to straighten the body and prevent crippling deformities. For the first time as well, surgery could be offered for the removal of cancerous tumors, where the careful dissection required could not possibly have been performed on the struggling patient of earlier eras.

19

Without the many diagnostic tools that are commonplace today, however, many patients would have been subjected to surgery, only to find their problems unresolved or perhaps even further complicated by the well-intentioned surgical intervention.

There is concern that some surgeons may be overly optimistic in recommendations for back surgery

Fortunately, with the modern technical advancement of noninvasive diagnostic resources available to surgeons today, including CAT scans, MRIs and PET scans, selection of patients can be much more carefully undertaken. It should be far less likely for a surgical procedure to be offered to a patient unless a positive outcome can be reasonably expected.

In the very best centers, this is truly the case. Some researchers in this field, however, have expressed concern that surgeons may be overly optimistic in their recommendations for back surgery, with a large group of patients still unsatisfied with their clinical improvement one year post-surgery.

With appropriately selected patients, modern surgery can offer replacement of degenerated intervertebral discs with artificial discs, as well as repair of collapsed and fractured osteoporotic vertebral bodies through procedures known as vertebroplasties. In this surgical procedure, the collapsed vertebra is reinflated with the injection of a fast-drying cement, restoring it to pre-fracture height and strength.

Although these new surgical therapies represent the cutting edge of science today, surgery, unfortunately, can only be offered as a solution to a relatively small percentage of the population suffering from back pain. Only 3% to 4% of patients with back pain will have attributable evidence suggesting surgical management could be helpful in improving their discomfort to a degree justifying operative intervention.

Understandably, every surgeon wants only the very best results. A collection of patients with "failed surgical back syndromes" can quickly stall any growing neurosurgical or orthopedic surgical practice, making the resultant chronic back care a significant and burdensome portion of the surgeon's daily workload.

Massage, Manual Therapies and Medicines: Ministrations in the Treatment of Back Pain

By default, the remaining non-surgical therapies used in the treatment of back pain are thereby unceremoniously lumped together under the all-encompassing umbrella of medical therapies.

This means that the 96% to 97% of back pain sufferers that cannot be treated with surgery, fall into the category in which their back pain will be treated—if treated at all—with *medical management strategies*. Some of these therapeutic modalities can be described as "mainstream" medical therapies, but the vast majority are known generally as Complementary or Alternative Medicines (CAM).

Massage is probably the oldest dated therapy in the treatment of back pain. Massage therapy likely began when the first human stumbled and fell and realized that by rubbing the injured limb they were able to significantly affect and improve the pain. Every major civilization since has incorporated massage into their healing arts. Today, many schools of practice exist throughout the world in the treatment of muscular pain including back pain.

Manual therapy is often differentiated from massage therapy, although many masseuses incorporate manual therapy in their practices. Manual therapy emphasizes therapeutic techniques, which not only involve treatment of the soft tissue inflammation, but also specifically address treatment methods designed to manipulate and mobilize affected joints in an effort to restore functional movement.

Like surgery, manual therapy techniques have been historically documented in the ancient medical literature. One of the earliest recorded images can be seen in this gruesome 16th-century woodcut image taken from Guido Guidi's textbook of medicine, illustrating traction applied to the spine, as described by Galen, one of the founders of Greek medicine. One can only imagine the obvious discomfort this patient must have suffered, to consent to treatment using an apparatus that was just as likely to have been found in a prison.

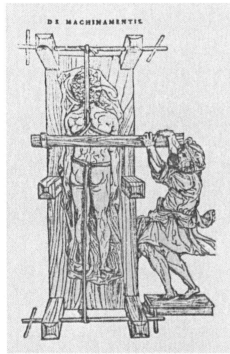

Application of spinal traction. From Guido Guidi's Chirurgia (16th century woodcut)

Over time, various schools of manual therapy in the different civilizations of man would craft manipulative therapies through trial and error, coming up with techniques remarkably similar for joint mobilization, soft tissue manipulation and spinal traction, all in the pursuit of relieving pain and improving mechanical function. Many of these manual therapy techniques were likely to have been documented in languages lost and, most probably, many others were documented in modern languages specific to their regional scientific community.

The role of manual therapy and joint manipulation in the English-speaking world had its first documented place in medical literature recorded in England in the 1800s. Known as Bone Setters, the early practitioners of this art secretively guarded their techniques as proprietary trade practices, more reminiscent of a guild society than a profession, but in time were inducted into the mainstream of medical practice, holding a solid place in the medical armamentarium of the mid-19th century

It would not be until 1892, however, and the foundation of osteopathic schools in America by Andrew T. Still, that a formalized approach to the study of spinal mechanics and treatment would be generally outlined and published—along with the establishment of osteopathic schools to instruct these practices to new graduates. This would be followed shortly thereafter by the development of chiropractic by Daniel Palmer in 1897. Together these two modalities of therapy would spread throughout the world into the present day where they continue to enjoy wide popularity amongst the large population suffering from back pain.

Associated with the teaching of medicine in university settings, physiotherapy would be developed for the management of orthopedic injuries, both in a supportive role to facilitate rehabilitation of post-surgical patients, as well as in a primary referral resource in the non-surgical treatment of musculoskeletal injuries. In addition to the use of modalities including ultrasound, electrotherapy and other similar applications, many physiotherapists have developed skills in manual therapy as well as acupuncture in the treatment of their patients.

Modern Medicine and the Treatment of Chronic Back Pain

Medical physicians today, although actively involved in the management of back pain, often find their traditional clinical role constrained to the prescription of medications, which are commonly prescribed in conjunction with referral to physiotherapists, chiropractors and masseuses who provide the traditional, supportive physical modalities of care.

Most medical pain-management specialists would agree that the vast majority of drugs prescribed by physicians in the treatment of back pain would be best described as palliative rather than curative. Palliative treatment describes a clinical management strategy directed towards pain management rather than the resolution of the underlying cause of the back pain.

23

In many cases of acute back pain, only a one- or two-week course of prescribed medicine may be required if the problem is self-limiting and following a natural history of eventual resolution. In other cases, however, the course of medical management would be better described as chronic, where the pattern of pain and disability persists, waxing and waning with each associated exacerbation and remission, but essentially continuing, unresolved.

In these cases, the underlying problem is ongoing and there is no known drug formulary to cure the problem. These patients, while under medical management, will probably have at least one pre-scribed medication in the treatment of the associated pain. It is also probable that the patient will be taking at least one other "non-prescribed", over-the-counter medication or nutraceutical, which their physician may, or perhaps may not, know about. Drug inter-actions can occur between all medications, including both pre-scribed and the complementary and alternative medications, and may be responsible for dangerous and, on rare occasions, fatal side effects.

Analgesics or painkillers are the most commonly prescribed drugs for treatment of back pain. They are a class of drugs that serve only one common purpose: reducing the sensory awareness of ex-perienced pain. These drugs as a class incorporate a wide spec-trum of medications, including acetylsalicylic acid (first sold by Bayer as Aspirin), acetaminophen (Tylenol), and many other vari-ous non-narcotic analgesics commonly used for pain.

The earliest effective painkiller in the history of medicine—and probably the most important drug ever introduced into the practice of medicine—was the family of narcotic drugs isolated from the opium poppy. The introduction of laudanum in early medicine, a narcotic extract isolated from the gum of the opium poppy, gave physicians the capability of bringing merciful comfort to the pa-tients charged to their care, even if there was precious little they could do to save a life or improve the course of a chronic, debilitat-ing illness.

Laudanum quickly became a popular favorite for the treatment of pain, as it provided not only a significantly decreased sensory awareness of the pain, but also a pleasingly enhanced mood. As it was commonly available and not closely regulated when first introduced, it is not surprising that there were those who were injudicious in their use of the drug, subsequently developing dependency problems with all the attendant risks that we unfortunately see in those afflicted in our society today.

There are many different narcotics presently on the market for the treatment of pain syndromes, including codeine, morphine, pethidine, oxycodone, hydromorphone, methadone and fentanyl. All are potent painkillers, but have their individual spectrum of unpleasant side effects, even when used with caution. One of the more common side effects experienced, involves the significant gastrointestinal side effects, including nausea, vomiting and constipation, often requiring additional concomitant prescriptions of laxatives and stool softeners, along with a high-fibre diet and necessary additional fluids.

Although not commonly recommended today for treatment of chronic, nonmalignant pain, including chronic back pain, narcotics are frequently prescribed for newly acute presentations of back pain, temporarily providing much-needed relief from the almost unbelievable agony. In cases where all other treatment appears to have failed, narcotics can, on occasion, also be used in the treatment of chronic, unremitting and disabling back pain syndromes.

The use of narcotics in treatment of chronic back pain syndromes, however, must always be tempered with the knowledge that they are also associated with cognitive impairment, which can often be missed by prescribing physicians, caregivers or even spouses, especially when used in older patients. This tendency towards cognitive impairment needs to be balanced with the consequences of the disability itself, which can also impede the ability to take care of oneself and establish functional independence. The decision to use narcotics for treatment of chronic back pain must only be taken after a careful assessment by the medical team responsible for care and management—and must be monitored judiciously to note any change in functional status.

Probably the most popular class of medications used in the treatment of back pain in the past 25 years, are grouped together in the pharmaceutical family called anti-inflammatories. The origin of this entire class of drugs stems from the discovery of the common aspirin, acetylsalicylic acid (ASA), a drug which was isolated from willow bark in the late 1800s and was long used by indigenous peoples in North America for treatment of pain syndromes.

> The vast majority of drugs prescribed in the treatment of back pain are palliative— not curative

In today's modern pharmacopoeia, not much has changed with derivatives from the same family of drugs widely found in every household in North America, available in both over-the-counter preparations and the more potent anti-inflammatory formularies prescribed by physicians for the treatment of back pain.

In spite of their widespread use, considerable debate as to their efficacy has existed in the medical community for some time. Little evidence is available to support their long-term effectiveness in addressing or resolving back pain. In addition to the lack of efficacy, there was considerable alarm in the medical community when overwhelming evidence came to light confirming that the widespread use of these medications was not only responsible for many deaths secondary to hemorrhage from gastrointestinal tracts, but may have been responsible, as well, for up to tens of thousands who succumbed to cardiovascular-related deaths in North America each year.

With publication of this bulletin, the culpable anti-inflammatories were abruptly withdrawn from the market, while medical researchers regrouped to assess the collateral damage.

There will no doubt be increased scrutiny and attention paid to the remaining anti-inflammatories on the market, as well as any future drugs that will be developed in this class, as there has certainly not been any clear benefit—at least when it comes to the treatment of chronic back pain.

Other drugs used in the palliative management of back pain are the various muscle relaxants, either by prescription or commonly available over-the-counter preparations. They are typically empirically formulated in combination with analgesics and, as such, their independent affect in the treatment of back pain is often difficult to assess.

One of the newer classes of pain management medications, originally developed for the treatment of epilepsy, are neuroleptics. On occasion, these may be specifically prescribed for treatment of chronic neuropathic pain syndromes manifesting as back pain. Unfortunately, only a very small segment of back pain patients are candidates for a trial of treatment using these drugs. Although not well tolerated in large dosages, this class of drug has been significantly successful in the treatment of selected patients, especially when other drugs have proved ineffective in the management of these markedly disabling neuropathic pain syndromes.

The CAM Therapies: Complementary and Alternative Medicines

If one describes *medications* generally, as any orally taken preparation, whether in liquid or tablet form, ingested for the purpose of treatment of back pain, then **medications** describe all other forms of medical therapies taken by mouth, including nutraceuticals, vitamins and the multitude of other proprietary preparations and formulations commonly used in the treatment of back pain.

It is not unreasonable to say that each of these recommended preparations and formulations, whether taken singularly or in conjunction with other preparations, has been temporarily successful, at least in part, in the alleviation of chronic back pain. In fact, most back sufferers will have historically made a decision to take one, if not several, of these preparations on the recommendation of a close friend or family member, based on anecdotal evidence.

In fact, much of the supporting evidence of these treatments would be described as "in vitro", indicating that whereas laboratory evidence may suggest a strong rationale for therapy, controlled clinical studies on people are less conclusive in support of their efficacy when subjected to the statistical rigors of modern scientific examination.

> Despite widespread use, the efficacy of anti-inflammatories is under considerable debate

In spite of the marginal evidence for use of medicines, both prescribed and non-prescribed, there remains a remarkable enthusiasm for these widely recommended therapies. One cannot help but be reminded of the observation penned by the famous physician, William Osler, when he wrote, "The desire to take medicine is perhaps the greatest single feature that distinguishes man from animals," written in 1925 while completing his biography of another famous Western physician, Harvey Cushing. We could only guess at how flabbergasted he would be if he were to examine the range of backache medicines commonly found in the modern medicine cabinet today.

It is not surprising then, with only a marginal success in the treatment of back pain attained by the mainstream medical establishment, that the doors have been flung open to find considerable enterprise exercised by many diverse practitioners of the healing arts, bringing forth the varied diverse therapies used in the treatment of the common backache today.

Physicians and surgeons specializing in the management and care of back pain provide some of these therapies, whereas alternatively credentialed healthcare practitioners instructed in the treatment of back problems and other musculoskeletal pain syndromes offer others. The instruction of some types of therapy may be less formalized, with the credentialing process less rigorous. Consequently, the individual skills and effectiveness of therapy may be

CAM Therapies
Used in the Treatment of Chronic Back Pain

Manual Therapies: Acupressure, Chiropractic, Cranial Sacral Therapy, Massage Therapy, Osteopathic Medicine, Physiotherapy, Reflexology, Reiki

Medical Therapies: Anthroposophic Medicine, Aromatherapy, Ayurvedic Medicine, Herbal Medicine, Homeopathy, Naturopathy, Traditional Chinese Medicine, Traditional Medical Practices

Invasive Medical Therapies: Acupuncture, Neural Acupuncture, Prolotherapy, Neural Therapy, Intramuscular Stimulation (IMS), Kolgavi Needling Technique

Exercise Therapies: Alexander Technique, Qi Gong, Taijiquan / Tai Chi, Yoga, Feldenkrais, Pilates, Schulz's Autogenic Training, Body / Mind Centering

Dietary Therapies: Nutritional Therapy, Special Diets, Vegetarian / Vegan Diets

perceived as appreciably different from one practitioner to another. Many of these modalities of therapy, however, have been practiced for generations. One can expect that they will continue as commonplace therapies only because of their intermittent success, providing a steady stream of enthusiastic supporters and new clientele. Even if science cannot explain the success of a specific therapy, as long as it continues to produce positive outcomes with sufficient enough frequency, new patients will be willingly encouraged to trial their services.

The enclosed table, although probably not inclusive, lists many of the popular CAM therapies applied in the management of chronic back pain. Many of these therapies are common and widespread, whereas others may be seen more rarely. In one form or another, most have been practiced for hundreds of years.

As a group, Complementary and Alternative Medicines (CAM) are defined today as an assemblage of diverse medical and healthcare systems, practices and products, not presently considered part of conventional medicine. They include a wide and sometimes confusing range of modalities and, when used in treatment of back pain, are often combined with each other, as well as with mainstream medicine.

The majority of back pain sufferers commonly express the belief that the use of complementary and alternative medicines together with conventional medicine is better than using either alone. As a consumer group, CAM users tend to be younger, well educated, with higher disposable incomes and often have wider social networks providing them with more diverse health information.

The evidence-based published results for most CAM therapies as previously noted, are often insufficient to draw firm conclusions about their efficacy and safety. As many of these therapies have only recently entered into the field of back pain management, it is important to remember that lack of evidence may not necessarily mean lack of efficacy, but rather that the therapy has not yet been adequately tested.

For the most part, mainstream medicine has voiced only grudging objection to CAM's intrusion into an area where modern medicine has been significantly lacking in effective solutions. Following the ancient Latin medical dictum immortalized in Hippocrates' oath, *"primum non nocere...above all, do no harm..."*, most of the CAM therapies are of a very low and likely acceptable risk, implying that it would be very unlikely that the patient would come out worse off after the treatment than before they had presented for care.

An obvious exception to this statement would include the invasive therapies, which involve specific risks directly related to needle placement. A wrongfully placed needle can result in immediate, serious consequences including sudden death. Additionally, many of the invasive therapies involve injections of drugs, all of which have their attendant risks of drug reactions and interactions including anaphylaxis, which may also result in sudden death.

The line between mainstream medicine and some of the more common CAM therapies has become blurred

The other therapeutic modalities that carry the risk of significant neurological compromise or death, are the various manual therapies as they are specifically used in the treatment of neck pain. There is a very rare but identifiable risk of stroke following manual therapies of the neck and it can occur regardless of the practitioner responsible for application of the treatment. As a group, physicians, osteopaths, chiropractors, physiotherapists and masseuses have all experienced these complications, which, although rare, have resulted in catastrophic outcomes. Put into perspective, the risk of experiencing a fatal complication from a manual therapy session of the neck is several hundred times less than that of experiencing a fatal complication from repeatedly using aspirin or anti-inflammatories given the very real risk of gastrointestinal bleeding and hemorrhage.

31

Over time, the lines between mainstream medicine and some of the more common CAM therapies have become somewhat blurred, with the general population perceiving many of them as already included in the mainstream treatment of back pain. It is not a useful exercise, however, to debate the various benefits and relative efficacies of the various treatments used in the management of back pain, for each of the therapies may be aimed at addressing different, specific contributing factors resulting in back pain. Because of the multifactorial etiology responsible for back pain syndromes, it would be equally erroneous to assume that any single therapy represents a panacea to the treatment of chronic back pain.

The Shortcomings of Chronic Back Pain Therapy Today

In general, the quality of the published back pain literature is not given the same general "sterling stamp" as is other integral areas of medical study and scientific publication. This is commonly attributed to the difficulty in achieving objective and reproducible measurement standards comparing results across different study protocols. Other arenas of medical research easily satisfy study methodology standards, thereby achieving acceptance by fellow scientists, as the results are easily measured, reproduced, and objectively agreed upon.

Examples of such objective findings include: controlled study survival rates to a specific treatment; objective scientific records comparing clinical measurements such as blood pressure, respiratory rates or urinary output; or standardized blood tests measuring drug levels or serum hormonal changes—all results of which can be standardized and serially documented.

When dealing with evaluation of pain syndromes or general scales of well-being, the objective markers are less exact, requiring some leeway for the individual participants in the study to provide subjective input to their study evaluators as to changes in quality, duration or intensity of pain, before and following application of various treatment modalities.

As soon as these subjective parameters come into play, considerable difficulty arises in evaluating common objectives—even when two parallel studies evaluate the same parameter. The scientific methodology of the study comes under intense criticism as many of these investigative trials are not designed with randomized, controlled groups or, perhaps, quantitative evaluation lacks heterogeneity of inclusion criteria and outcome definitions. All of these parameters must be carefully evaluated in determining the quality of research as they aid the reviewer in deriving conclusions that can be readily accepted and agreed upon by other discerning reviewers.

> Readers of this book are likely to have tried at least two or more different therapies in the search for back pain relief

All of the modalities of therapy in treatment of back pain have enjoyed some success. Clearly, no therapy will continue to exist, often for generations, without at least some marginal success. In fact, most people who are reading this book will have trialed at least two, if not more, of these various therapies in search of a solution for existing pain, including chronic low back pain.

What the research does tends to support is the premise that many—if not most—of these therapies, although demonstrating an initial positive response, are less likely to have documented, substantial residual improvement at one-year post treatment. They almost all require an ongoing treatment protocol for maintenance of the improvement, a situation that is often discouraging to the chronic back pain sufferer who experiences the indignity of the attendant loss of empowerment and dependency upon one or more therapists to maintain a level of comfort.

Many of the therapies utilized in the treatment of back pain have one thing in common: they address the problem of the patient in a passive manner, applying the treatment to the patient, with no significant input required in return from the patient in the treatment solution of the back pain. And, as patients, that is exactly the type of ideal solution that we are seeking. Why expend any personal time or effort to resolve a problem if unnecessary?

It would appear, however, that something else is required in the formula to improve the predictability of success in the treatment of chronic back pain. The clue to the puzzle may lie in the evidence that suggests a combination of modalities, especially when exercise is included in the treatment mix, is most likely to result in sustained improvement.

In addition, most back pain experts would agree that the type of exercise is probably not as important as the frequency of the exercise, daily exercise being the ideal prescription. Considerable study into the effects of exercise supports the premise that exercise provides several benefits in the rehabilitation of the chronic back pain syndrome, with improvements in core strength and balance most likely the contributing paramount influence. This prescription equally applies to almost all chronic back pain syndromes, regardless of their origin.

It may also be true that the rehabilitation and implementation of simple ergonomic postural corrections may be the single most important part of the exercise program contributing to the improvement in core strength and balance and the eventual improvement in chronic backache.

This is good news indeed! For whatever the cause of our chronic back pain and misery, there is something that is easily achievable.

Lying within the grasp of each of us is the opportunity every day to improve our posture and garner the resultant pain-relieving benefits.

Understanding and Recognizing Postural Chronic Back Pain

4

Posture: *the recognizable upright stance that describes, and is a result of, the overall synthesis of the positions of all the body's weight-bearing joints at any "point of time". It may be a habitual position developed "overtime", or a specific position taken during a given activity.*

The ideal postural stance is probably best seen in young, healthy children, when the center of gravity runs perfectly through the central axis of the body, with little need for thought, care or attention. In perfect upright posture, the center of gravity consistently runs through recognizable skeletal landmarks as demonstrated in the accompanying diagram on the next page.

The clinical examination of posture and assessment of misalignments and imbalances can be accurately assessed by therapists using backdrop grid boards and plumb lines to examine the symmetry of bony landmarks and joint positions in a bilateral comparison. When required, these assessments can be done serially throughout a therapeutic program to confirm progress as evidenced by measurements of changing landmarks.

The assessment of this *gravitational axis line* is quite simple to understand and put into practice. The term gravitational axis line describes an imaginary vertical line running through the erect body, in which the weight of the torso, including the head and neck, is balanced both in front and behind, as well as from one side to the other.

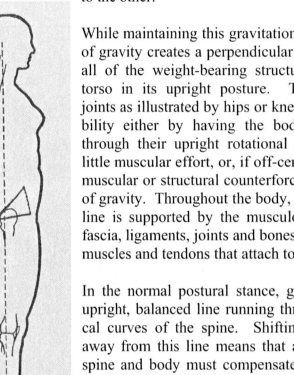

While maintaining this gravitational axis line, the force of gravity creates a perpendicular vector stress through all of the weight-bearing structures that support the torso in its upright posture. These weight-bearing joints as illustrated by hips or knees, maintain their stability either by having the body mass fall exactly through their upright rotational axis, which requires little muscular effort, or, if off-center, by maintaining a muscular or structural counterforce to offset the effects of gravity. Throughout the body, this gravitational axis line is supported by the musculoskeletal elements of fascia, ligaments, joints and bones, and is moved by the muscles and tendons that attach to these structures.

In the normal postural stance, gravity acts upon this upright, balanced line running through the physiological curves of the spine. Shifting the body's weight away from this line means that another region of the spine and body must compensate to regain a postural equilibrium and stability.

The Different Types of Aberrant Posture

There are many anatomical deformities that can contribute to an altered centerline of gravity and postural malalignment. Many of these we may have been born with, whereas others will have been acquired along the way following injuries or diseases that may affect the metabolism, development or formation of the musculoskeletal system. Some of these causes may be as obvious as a congenital scoliosis or curvature of the spine, which will affect us throughout the course of our life, or, less obviously, flat feet, which will cause excessive outward pronation at the ankles and a compensatory twisted pelvis. These causes will produce, in spite of the body's best efforts, a fixed anatomical end-point impingement preventing the body from achieving the normally erect physiological gravitational axis line.

Surprisingly enough, there is very little discomfort directly associated with these postural anomalies, especially if they occur from birth or early on in life, when the body has been given the opportunity to accommodate to these changes during the growing and developmental phase.

More commonly, however, the postural malalignments not due to these previously described, underlying, early-life anatomical deformities are secondary to loss of core strength from multiple causes with an eventual loss of neurological kinesthetic awareness in the maintenance of normal equilibrium and balance.

Basically, there are two distinct types of postural aberration, one being far more common than the other. In the early medical texts of the 1900s, dating back to the time of the "posture police" in the last century and the popular posture clinics, these two variants of postural malalignment were termed *"gorilla"* and *"kangaroo"*. Neither of these two terms was very flattering, perhaps reflecting an arrogance of the attending physician in those times when bedside manner may not have been of the import and expectation that it is today.

The more common postural abnormality, which was called the "gorilla posture", is identified with the center of gravity being displaced forward. Much less common is the "kangaroo posture", which describes the centerline of gravity being displaced backward, with the pelvis almost seeming to lead the movement forward.

In both of these situations, the disturbance of equilibrium with displacement of the axial gravitational line creates an unanticipated physiological stress on all of the weight-bearing joints, including ankles, knees and hips, pelvic girdle and spinal column. The excessive and prolonged demands placed upon the involved muscles and joints supporting the spine cause fatigue and inflammation of the supporting muscles, stress on fascia and ligaments and deformity of joint capsules—all physiological factors contributing to the inflammatory patterns recognized as chronic postural back pain.

The Gorilla Posture Model

The forward type of posture abnormality is identified with the image of shoulders drooping forward and rounding to the front, with the chin tilting upward. The lower dorsal and lumbar curves are less defined and the axial line of the lower dorsal and lumbar curves slants downward and backward. The front of the pelvis is tipped forward and is associated with weakening of the frontal abdominal musculature.

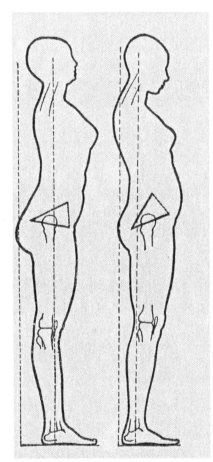

Kangaroo   Gorilla

In the days of early Victorian fashion, this type of posture was often caused by core muscle atrophy secondary to corset pressure. The corset produced the desired effect of the slender, hourglass-tapering waist, but, unfortunately, at the cost of pushing down and producing the associated broad and excessively padded hips, a deformity caused by the combined effect of tight lacing and insufficient exercise.

Today, this type of postural abnormality commonly occurs with fatigue from any cause, a posture we have all assumed at one time or another, when shuffling forward with each step seems easier than the effort necessary to stand upright and pick up our feet when walking.

The Gorilla posture commonly occurs with fatigue from any variety of causes

The changed gravitational axis is now displaced forward to the front of the hip joints, producing stretching of the hamstrings and an indolent relaxation of the hip flexors. The knees are displaced backward into hyperextension, and the center of gravity moves to the front of the knee joint. This forces the weight of the body to be anterior of the mid-foot, with the strain pushing forward onto the ball of the planted foot.

The Kangaroo Posture Model

Seen much less frequently, this type of postural abnormality is identified by the head tilting downward and the shoulders being back of the central line of gravity. The axial gravitational line of the lower dorsal and lumbar spine is slanted forward and the sacrum is tilted backward, creating additional strain on the sacroiliac joints.

This center of gravity is displaced to the back of the hip joint, creating a tension on the front of the body where the ilio-psoas, abdominal muscles and flexor muscle group of the hips, strain to keep the body upright. The knees are forward of the center axis and the weight of the body now rests backward of the mid-foot, sitting back on the heels. This creates an increased tension pattern in the front muscles of the lower legs as they try to stabilize the posteriorly displaced center of gravity.

With this simple understanding of the basic bioengineering principles involved in the physiological evolution of erect posture, it is not difficult to recognize these two types of aberrant posture. It is also not difficult to understand why aberrant posture causes the symptoms we recognize as chronic postural back pain.

The Acute Back Pain Syndrome: How Acute Back Pain Is Different from Postural Chronic Back Pain

The following general explanations and diagnoses are often used when physicians or therapists explain the etiology of this pattern of chronic back pain to the unfortunate owner.

1. normal wear and tear
2. natural aging of bone and joint
3. loss of core fitness
4. poor ergonomic positioning
5. mechanical backache
6. biomechanical backache
7. chronic, non-specific back pain
8. degenerative osteoarthritis

The acute back pain syndrome is a type of back pain that is not easily forgotten, and very unlikely to be confused with chronic postural backache. It is characterized by significant, acute muscle spasm—the kind that keeps you quite bent over if it is affecting your low back, encouraging very careful execution of movements, gingerly ensuring that nothing further aggravates this exceptionally exquisite pain.

The origin of this acute spasm may be secondary to trauma: either a direct blow or strain causing an inflammation process in the myofascial tissues themselves or a secondary splinting phenomena, with the muscles guarding an underlying injured structure. This can occur, for example, in the presence of a ruptured disk in its acute stages, fractures of the underlying spine or other significant events, all of which create symptoms that are easily differentiated from the patterns of chronic postural backache.

Fortunately, acute back pain is almost always brought to a physician's attention, as the pain is generally severe enough to warrant prescriptions for narcotic analgesics. A proper examination and investigation at the time of presentation will almost always reveal the underlying cause, at which time the options for appropriate treatment can be considered.

The Four Classical Key Points that Distinguish Chronic Postural Back Pain

If you have chronic postural back pain, more than likely the following clinical picture is a fairly accurate description of your medical case history.

1. You may have dated the onset of your back pain to events that signal overuse, strain or mild trauma, or you will have found that the symptoms just gradually came on, with no specific etiology responsible.
2. The back pain will generally be localized to the soft-tissue areas aligning the spine and may be associated with radiation to the back of the shoulder and pelvic girdle areas. On occasion it may radiate to the arms and legs, but rarely more distally than the knees or elbows. It will not be accompanied by any motor loss or specific muscle weakness indicative of a neurological deficit.
3. Your back pain will have been present for several months or more, generally waxing and waning in severity depending on your day-to-day activities. And although you think it may have drastically changed your life, you feel otherwise well and the back pain has not been associated with any other significant deterioration in your general health.
4. You will probably have visited your physician and investigations including MRI, CAT scan, x-ray and bloodwork will not have demonstrated any serious or significant medical condition requiring either surgical or medical intervention.

Some of these terms are pseudonyms used in description of idiopathic or non-specific chronic back-pain syndrome. Other terms describe radiological changes that may accompany the chronic back-pain syndrome but may not be directly responsible for the accompanying pain. Still others describe problems that would best be considered secondary diagnoses, their onset developing later in the timeline of postural back pain and reflecting a loss of musculoskeletal function—changes that come about when we make alterations in our physical activities and lifestyle in response to the presence of chronic pain.

An insidious path describes the origin and course of postural back pain. Because there may not be a significant, identifiable event resulting in the onset of the pain syndrome, chronic postural back pain is more likely to be associated with overwork, repetitive activities, fatigue or an underlying minor injury—or even stress. Unless the initial back-pain episode is markedly severe, there is not generally a significant concern at first, as postural back pain, although debilitating over time, is rarely severe enough to leave a person bedridden.

The more weight we gain and the more fitness we lose, the more likely the onset of back pain

There is also a tendency to believe that postural back pain will probably get better on its own. For this reason it is often neglected for some time prior to the decision to see a doctor or therapist for care. There may also be the tendency to ignore the nagging back pain as a natural aging process, accepting the level of disability as being part and parcel of moving into middle age.

In spite of an extended period of aggravation, embarrassment may additionally delay evaluation and treatment. Most of us recognize that our weight and level of fitness are not what they had been in earlier years and within ourselves we recognize that these factors are a contributing factor to our ongoing disability—and without doubt, this is true. The more weight that we gain and the more fitness that we lose, the more likely we will be plagued by the onset of postural backache.

We who number among these, however, should take heart in the knowledge that even being "horizontally challenged" does not mean that significant improvement in pain and quality-of-life cannot be gained by taking some simple steps to improve our postural alignment.

The Myth of Spinal Osteoarthritis and Chronic Back Pain

Many people believe that chronic back pain is synonymous with the aging process, especially when it is pointed out to them that their x-rays or MRIs demonstrate evidence of degenerative osteoarthritis.

It would be a significant error in judgment to come to this conclusion for two very important reasons. The first, it is relatively uncommon to find spinal films, after a person reaches the age of 40, that do not demonstrate some element of degenerative osteoarthritis; and, in fact, osteoarthritis is commonly found much earlier in life, especially when there has been an antecedent history of trauma or injury. The second, and far more important, finding is that the significant majority of people in whom these degenerative changes can be demonstrated have absolutely no symptoms of backache.

Although osteoarthritis can be a significant cause of disability and joint pain, especially when involving the large weight-bearing joints like hips and knees, it generally is not a common cause of back pain. That is not to say that osteoarthritic joints in the spine cannot be painful. They most certainly can, especially if subjected to torsional trauma such as a whiplash injury or if they become inflamed from the effects of a *weekend-warrior overuse syndrome*; but a non-arthritic, normal joint would very likely demonstrate a similar inflammatory pattern under the same circumstances.

Many people confuse osteoarthritis with the other group of distinctive disabling and painful *inflammatory arthropathies*. These diseases, characterized by the examples of rheumatoid arthritis, lupus erythematosus or gout, present with painfully swollen, hot and inflamed joints. Markedly different in presentation, osteoarthritis can be a relatively benign event with few if any symptoms.

Postural chronic back pain can be present when spinal x-rays are normal

Osteoarthritis is, however, associated with morphological changes in the joint cartilage, which covers and lines the surface of all synovial joints. Fissures as well as pits and grooves form in the previously smooth cartilage surface and are identified as recognizable, degenerative changes of osteoarthritis.

In the spine, the joints affected by this osteoarthritis are called apophyseal joints, pairs of joints existing on each side of individual vertebral bodies. The apophyseal joints create articulations joining each vertebral body to the one above and below it. It is the free movement of these apophyseal joints that allow the head and neck, as well as the rest of the spine. to swivel multi-dimensionally on its axis. These joints allow movement that includes side bending, flexion, extension and twisting, all complex motions that give the spine its graceful movement comparable to twirling a string of pearls.

Development of osteoarthritic changes in these apophyseal joints may, over time, result in obstruction to the previously enjoyed gliding movement and interfere with the normal, expected range of motion. This measurable interference in loss of normal spinal range of motion may be associated with chronic postural back pain, but may not necessarily be a causative factor, for chronic postural back pain can be present when spinal x-rays are absolutely normal, without any evidence of osteoarthritis.

What Causes the Symptoms of Chronic Back Pain?

Several causative mechanisms come into play in the production of the symptoms of postural back pain. The entire process begins with deviation of the spine from its normal physiological gravitational axis into one of the variant malalignment postures. Maintaining this aberrant position for an extended period of time results in uncharacteristic mechanical stresses on the well-innervated joint capsules and ligaments, as well as mechanical irritation of the receptive sensory nerve endings within the supporting muscles themselves.

This pain pattern, termed "nociceptive" after the root term *noxious*, is initially felt in local tissues subjected to the persistent and prolonged stretch, but later will become more generalized and widespread as adjacent muscles take up some of the effort to assist in minimizing the increasing strain. Reducing the mechanical stress placed on the affected structures, by changing position or performing a different activity, usually improves and may perhaps even dissipate this type of pain completely.

Overtime, if these postural imbalances persist, a contralateral adaptive shortening of the muscles and fascia occurs in response to the stretched tissues occurring locally as well as elsewhere in the structural musculoskeletal system. This adaptive shortening of spinal curves occurs in the process of stabilizing the body's newly acquired posture against the altered central axis of gravity. The same muscles and fascia may also shorten if rehabilitation is neglected following trauma, surgery or prolonged inactivity, such as enforced bed rest, and understandably becomes the focus of attendant therapy in these cases.

After a period of weeks and months with this new posture, further pain can be attributed to the stress placed on these pathologically shortened tissues. This evolving process of the combined tissue stretching and the compensatory tissue shortening creates visibly evident postural dysfunctional patterns that are major contributors to the symptoms underlying postural back pain.

Associated with the presence of this dysfunctional movement pattern, is a recognizable, asymmetrical tension in the supporting musculature surrounding the regional spinal column. This tension pattern in the affected muscles is almost always tender to touch and palpation, and a recognizable contribution to postural back pain. The presence of this increased myofascial tension is the body's reaction to a shift off the normally vertical gravitational axis, as it must now increase its efforts to support the newly positioned body against the gravitational forces in this new ergonomically compromised position. This increased workload, with the attendant production of irritant lactic acid (a by-product of muscle metabolic activity) and progressive, painful nociceptive nerve stimulation, results in the sensory overload that we interpret as chronic back pain.

The quality and intensity of postural chronic back pain tends to fluctuate throughout the day

The quality and intensity of the pain caused by postural backache tends to wax and wane throughout the course of the day, dependent on workload and specific tasks, the level of associated fatigue and even the time of day. In general, although often accompanied by a period of stiffness, mornings are generally best. Later on in the day, as we get more fatigued, the discomfort tends to increase. The back pain will generally improve if we can put up our feet and, better yet, if we can lie down—even for a short rest.

46

Following someone with chronic postural back pain and plotting the imaginary gravitational axis line running through their spine during the course of the day will easily demonstrate the affect of fatigue on the alteration of spinal column alignment, as the center of gravity shifts toward the weakened ergonomic posture. The overworking musculoskeletal system attempting to stabilize the errant spinal column will, in time, exhibit symptoms caused by the fatigued contractile component of the supporting musculature.

Chronic postural back pain is almost always accompanied by a general feeling of stiffness in the supporting musculature, notably following periods of being in one position for too long. After a night's sleep, it is common to feel stiff in the morning until one gets moving. The stiffness can occur in the same way following prolonged periods of sitting and is especially noted when moving from a sitting to a standing position, where several steps may be required before one feels comfortable being completely upright.

Correcting Postural Problems

Understanding chronic postural back pain is one thing, correcting a long-standing postural problem is quite another! As pointed out by the memorable American author Mark Twain, "I reckon just saying it don't make it so."

Although a thorough and complete examination by our attending physician, chiropractor or therapist reassures us that there is no significant underlying structural abnormality, this provides little solace with the realization that we are going to wake up to the same picture every morning unless something can be brought to bear to effect a change in the natural history of what everyone shrugs and accepts as a downhill course.

The good news is that there is something that can be done to improve the problem, regardless of how long it has been around. True enough, the shorter the history, the faster the response—but even in intransigent cases, improvement in symptoms can be realized within short weeks of paying attention to posture.

Understanding and Recognizing Postural Back Pain

All that is required is the understanding of a few simple "turn-key" principles and the resolve to keep them current in the stream of our consciousness, as often as we can throughout the course of the day. Within time, they will become ingrained as the new reality.

Moving Towards Perfect Posture

5

How Posture Is a Barometer of Health

Perfect posture is an elusive ideal that assumes we all possess normal textbook anatomy. Given the whole host of orthopedic anomalies, including flat feet, bowed legs, knocked knees, torqued pelvises due to short leg syndrome, dysfunctional movement patterns of sacroiliac joints, as well as the common scoliotic anomalies of the spine, it is not surprising to find a wide variation in the physical postural challenges faced by modern men and women.

If we have been injured along the way, with skeletal fractures, acceleration/deceleration injuries caused by whiplash, sporting collisions and other strains, or degenerative changes associated with aging, we will again be forced off the mark of achieving the classic, ideal posture.

For this very reason, it is likely flawed to believe, as many of us do (including some therapists), that each of us can be fitted to a preconceived mold of perfect posture. This is much like the golf or tennis instructor who tries to mold each student into the perfect swing or serve as dictated by the laws of physics, without consideration of age, flexibility or physical stature.

It is also important to remember that body posture is influenced by more than the mere expression of anatomy and physical energy. Postural stance reveals not only our genetic and social heritage, but collectively represents the accumulated mental and physical habits that we have taken a lifetime to gather. In addition, posture is a constantly changing yardstick reflecting our internal psychological status. This continuous flux influences and affects the ever-changing general physiological state we interpret as health and well being.

Ultimately, posture can be a barometer of our overall health

So, in the end, posture can also be a barometer of our overall health, dependent on the healthy functioning of many different control systems in our body. We take this all for granted, forgetting what a finely tuned instrument we are. Maintaining erect posture requires an intact, functioning central nervous system, a working visual system to orientate us to the horizon, and an operational vestibular system responsible for maintaining balance. Also critical to maintaining our posture are the various neurological sensors called proprioreceptors located throughout our musculoskeletal system, which tell us, even with our eyes closed, the position of each of our joints, whether our fingers are spread apart or held together, or whether we are about to sprain an ankle because we stepped on a small pebble and can feel the twisting stress in the supporting ligaments.

The system can work the other way as well. Not only is posture affected by the state and health of various control systems, changes in posture can trigger internal changes to come about within the body itself. Illustrations of this corollary are the changes in confidence and physical strength of which we become aware, having unconsciously straightened up, held our carriage erect, prepared to face an unexpected situation requiring that we take charge and rise to the occasion of a challenging circumstance. The more erect carriage allows our heart and lungs to work more effectively and the changes in spinal alignment increase our physical power, all transformations to which our internal monitoring systems immediately become aware and respond.

The Reality of "Practical" Posture

Ultimately, most of us adopt a compromised posture, a practical pose struck somewhere short of ideal or perfect. It is a weakness within us all that, given any excuse, we will slack off rather than give maximum effort. It is also the reason why we ask the inevitable question, "What's in it for me?"

Most of us will not willingly expend energy in directions that will not give us, if not immediate gratification, at least some reasonably expected satisfactory goal within the near future. We will do that which makes us feel better, especially if we do not have to expend much effort in attaining it. Most of us, given the opportunity, will be predictably self-serving. As one wise philosopher put it after years of careful study, "In all things, I do that which pleases me, so that in the end, at least one of us will be satisfied."

So "practical posture" is as good a place as any to begin this journey towards "perfect posture." It fits the style of "everything in moderation, including moderation." This tenet presupposes that we will pursue the goal of perfect posture with honest effort for a reasonable period of time. If it proves beneficial, we will continue the effort; if not, we will chose another path, dropping the first, like other blind alleys we may have gone down in the course of life. That probably reflects the philosophy of life a practical person would adhere to—most likely as good as we are going to get for effort!

> Things can be better than they are, if only we put some small steps into place

It also grants us some leeway to break the 100% rule and slip out of the mold occasionally, when we are tired or fatigued or just plain irritated with life around us.

At the same time, being practical people, we feel reasonably convinced that the principles of perfect posture are sound. If we give it just a little more effort, sticking with it just a wee bit longer, there may just be significant benefits that will make the trouble of all this worthwhile.

The Journey to Perfect Posture

The journey to perfect posture is all about expediency. We recognize that there may be extra effort required to overcome the inertia. We are also convinced, perhaps from past experience or practical knowledge, that things can be better than they are, if only we put some small steps into place. This may be no more difficult than keeping some simple stepping-stones to postural alignment a bit more visible in our "minds eye", with greater intensity and focus.

Like every great coach and trainer, the gifted exercise therapist challenged with the rehabilitation of a defective posture finds a communicative tool that allows them to relate to their client or patient, suggesting and building the kinesthetic clues necessary to create the concept of perfect posture from within. By taking this approach, the ideal concept of posture for that specific individual can take shape. As our intellect grapples with the offered visual conceptualization, our body responds to the kinesthetic clues and we move toward the model we have created in our mind.

Accompanying this posture program is a standard core-strength exercise routine to help overcome the fatigue of the supporting musculature required to maintain normal posture as the day progresses.

Perfect posture is a dynamic equilibrium, changing from moment to moment. With each movement, a delicate balance is created, surrounding our center of gravity. When executed perfectly, no muscle group is overly taxed as the body performs this marvelous neurological interplay between proprioceptive sensory input from our joints and muscles, conveying to the deep recesses of the brain our exact position relative to space and time, constantly instructing our muscles to ease or increase tension in the performance of this physiological ballet.

The concept of balance and posture remains a constant challenge to even the most elite dance artists, gymnasts and sport athletes as they strive for perfection. There can be no doubt that balance and posture contribute appreciably to the success of every elite athlete, as any sports fan can attest, having watched the dominance of Wayne Gretzky, Magic Johnson, and Tiger Woods in their respective fields. Every great ballet diva that has ever graced the stage has, as well, challenged the ethereal limits of balance and posture, engaging breathless audiences with the phenomenal poses of their art, as if nothing but air supported them.

Yin: a state of relaxation, rest and repair

Yang: a position of energy anticipatory of purposeful movement

Every one of these athletes recognizes that this journey to posture perfection starts from within—an embryo of an idea that develops and is transformed in a kinesthetic exchange resulting in the intentional movement executed by the body. While it is true that physical training is a critical part of this journey, ensuring that the physiological standards have been achieved in strengthening the core musculature, it is, in the end, the conceptualization of the postural model that begins the movement or pose.

How Chinese Medicine Paved the Way

Very few athletic pursuits have had as much work, research, and understanding in the theory of "rootedness" and posture as those related to the ancient Chinese martial arts. The study and theoretical contributions of the great Qigong and Taijiquan (Tai Chi) masters date back some three thousand years. Many of the classical writings from this ancient era have survived into modern literature with English translation by contemporary masters and dedicated students who have introduced Eastern martial arts into Western cultures. These writings may very possibly be the oldest documented studies of posture in civilization, where kinesthetic conceptual tools were the primary teaching methods.

Chinese medicine and the associated movement forms of Taijiquan and Qigong are formulated around the basic concepts of Yin and Yang. In terms of posture and movement, Yin and Yang have specific meanings. Yin is a state of relaxation, rest and repair, whereas Yang is a position of energy, anticipatory of purposeful movement. The flow of life energy or Qi (Chi) follows this pattern of balance, moving between rest and purposeful action, with balanced pairs of meridians supporting each of these two necessary facets of life.

The theories of posture and rootedness are taught to martial arts students with varying levels of complexity. The purpose of rootedness is to ensure that the combatant stays on his feet because the warrior that has been thrown or knocked to the ground is placed at great peril. Since the martial artist is most often in a position of standing alone on one leg, with the unweighted leg posed for use as a weapon, the concepts of balance and rootedness create great challenges.

In Chinese medicine, the complicated system of meridian pathways control the flow of energy or Qi as it flows over the entire surface and interior of the body, ensuring that the functions of the internal organs continue unimpeded, as well as defending the outside surface of the body from invasive challenges. Each of these meridians has many acupuncture points or entry gates for energy exchange and each acupuncture point is specifically designated as an active treatment point to either reinforce these defensive mechanisms or treat existing abnormalities of the interior organs. In total, there exist over 1,400 acupuncture points that can be used for treatment.

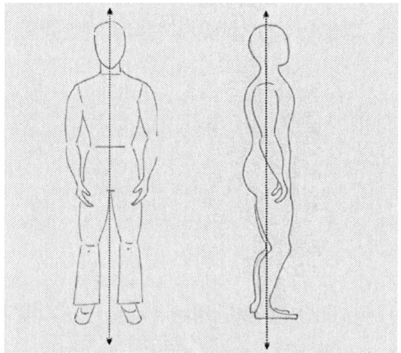

Qigong Wuji Position "The Great Emptiness"

The martial art student is encouraged through proprioceptive and kinesthetic clues to experience the flow of Qi energy as it courses through these meridians and energy gates in provision of the powerful stances required to carry out the actions of defense and attack.

The very first task in the study of erect posture is to understand and appreciate the first position, known as Wuji, describing a position of rest and point of neutrality. Translated into English from Chinese literature as "the great emptiness" or "the great nothingness", Wuji describes a pose midway between the two polarities of Yin and Yang. In the Chinese philosophy and appreciation of the duality of Yin/Yang, Wuji describes an almost indivisible point where the differentiation between Yin and Yang becomes infinitesimal.

Wuji refers to an erect posture of equilibrium, which may be described as the most balanced and relaxed posture that can exist midway between the states of Yin and Yang .Although relaxed, this postural position is also charged with anticipation, with the full capability of moving with commitment to either a Yin or Yang position. This pivotal state of balance is so delicate that martial art masters have described it as a state of balance within the body so fine that "if a butterfly were to alight on the person, it could be enough to set the body in motion towards either a Yin or Yang posture."

> Taijiquan is described as a ballet of opposites, with a ceaseless shifting between two polarities

Balanced posture in martial arts as in other athletic pursuits is not a fixed entity and is best described as a dance rather than a march. To be truly balanced in the Wuji state, there can be no tension or strain in the posture. The joints themselves must feel in the position of neutrality without tension in the ligaments or muscles controlling them. Any tension will result in the restriction of the flow of Qi and impede the stability of the stance.

Having learned the Wuji position, the martial art student's proprioceptive and kinesthetic appreciation is further challenged as the Taijiquan form moves off the neutral Wuji position towards either a Yin or Yang postural stance. Taijiquan is described as a ballet of opposites, with a ceaseless shifting between the two polarities. The movement in the form is a circular energy force compared with the spiral movement of a "string of pearls" and described in Taijiquan writings as "rooted in the foot, sprouted through the leg, governed at the waist and manifested in the fingers."

Visualizing Perfect Posture is Half the Battle

In moving toward this perfect postural stance, we too will face similar challenges as we search for that natural and supportive stance. Translating this kinesthetic experience in a meaningful way requires creative application. While it is helpful to work with a trained exercise therapist, with the benefit of mirrors and constant feedback in the study of our postural alignment, the reality dictates that, to achieve the goals of postural alignment, we must develop an inner sense of correct postural alignment.

Recognizing that each of us has our own physical imperfections, we must also realize that it is impossible for most of us to fit into the mold of perfect posture. Perfect posture must be individualized, allowing our inherent capabilities to arise from within like the fabled Phoenix, to facilitate the achievement of an individualized best-balanced posture. We are not all gazelles and, fortunately, we are also not all hippopotamuses; but for each of us, given the anatomy that we have inherited or acquired, there is a balanced postural carriage that will minimize the muscular forces required to hold us up against this axis of gravity. This can only be achieved through kinesthetic conceptualization, the process of directing our minds to conceive what it is that we wish our body to do and then allowing our body to move into the space and mold created by our mind.

Most of us, being aware of our poor posture at one time or another, have given ourselves "a mental kick in the pants" with admonishments to straighten up. Although we make an immediate effort to place ourselves in a better postural stance, it feels uncomfortable and contrived. The reason that it feels unnatural is that we are attempting to force our body into better postural carriage by consciously contracting certain muscles in an attempt to "pull" the body into what we conceive as normal postural alignment. Because of this strained cooperation between body and spirit, the effort is taxing and quickly abandoned as our train of thought changes. To find perfect posture, we have to have a different approach. Finding an improved natural postural carriage requires changing the paradigm, thinking not about forcing the mold onto the body, but rather creating change from within, conceptualizing and then "casting" the new postural stance.

Not so difficult to do, you say! Well, frankly, in the beginning you will be surprised at how often you will catch yourself slipping away from what just a moment ago, you promised yourself you would start paying attention to. There is no point in beating yourself up in frustration over these all-too-frequent initial lapses of concentration. It is expected, for at first the entire concept will be below our radar screen; but soon this will change. For now, just catch yourself and carry on.

Before you realize it, you will find that what seemed impossible to achieve at first has now become a habit. Your body will intuitively know when you are slipping out of postural alignment and provide you with the kinesthetic clues needed to help you correct yourself. Soon even this process will fall under the radar of consciousness. What once was a chore is no longer an effort. Within a very reasonable time, you will find yourself empowered by these efforts, reaping the benefits and well on your way to a more comfortable existence.

The 7 Red Flags of Back Pain

6

A Catalogue of Back Pain Pathology

Fostering alarm and having everyone's heart push into their throat is never a very good idea, but no discussion of back pain is complete without mention of these very important causes of back pain.

The rare causes of back pain to be discussed in this chapter must first be put into perspective: *only 3% to 4% of all back pains will be caused by any significant pathology.* Even if you have one of the diagnoses that you read about in this section, it is not necessarily reason to panic. Most are not inevitably catastrophic and medical therapy, in many cases, can effectively alter the course of the disease. Other causes in this list can even be quickly and permanently resolved with surgical intervention.

In the majority of these problems, however, it is important to make the diagnosis promptly and begin the appropriate medical care as soon as possible to reduce complications and bring about the best possible solution. So, if the symptoms in this section are descriptive of your current health condition, you must take the first step by presenting yourself to competent care for examination to rule out the presence of any significant disease, and begin treatment as required.

A proper examination and a high index of suspicion will almost always result in the attending physician ordering the appropriate studies to come up with an accurate diagnosis and proper therapy.

The catalogued list of pathological causes of back pain in the included table comprises a wide variety of problems that can be associated with back pain. This listing should not be considered an absolute register of possible pathological entities, as there will always be the exceptional aberrant presentation of back pain, which, although very rarely seen, will present in an uncharacteristic manner creating diagnostic dilemmas for attending physician and specialist alike. The group of diseases listed, however, does represent the most likely etiologies responsible for pathological back pain requiring medical or surgical intervention.

> One good thing about back pain: the longer you have had it—especially if it hasn't changed much—the more likely it is benign

When to Be Worried and When Not to Be Worried

There is one good thing about chronic back pain: the longer that you have had it, especially if it has not changed much, the more likely it is to be benign and not be included in this cluster of pathology. Almost all of the these diagnoses will present with back pain that is not pathogenomic or characteristic of the chronic back pain we have been discussing throughout this book, and will feature one or more of the symptoms listed under the 7 Red Flags.

The severity of the back pain is also not necessarily a good marker of how likely it is to fall into this group. Although the acute back pain syndrome described earlier can herald as one of these serious illnesses, more often, the acute back pain syndrome is unlikely to be associated with a sinister outcome. In fact, some of the most decidedly acute, painful presentations of back pain will respond surprisingly well to an intramuscular injection of narcotic medication, with the afflicted sufferer *"nodding off into the arms of Morphea"* and waking up several hours later, markedly improved. Pain tolerance also varies widely from person to person—a factor

The Pathological Causes of Back Pain

Cancers
Epidural or vertebral body cancer metastases
Multiple myeloma
Lymphoma
Primary epidural or intradural tumors

Inflammatory disorders
Ankylosing spondylitis
Psoriatic arthritis
Polymyalgia rheumatica
Reiter's syndrome and other reactive spondyloarthropathies
Primary fibromyalgia

Infections
Vertebral osteomyelitis
Epidural abscess
Discitis
Tuberculosis
Bacterial endocarditis
General sepsis

Metabolic diseases
Osteoporosis
Osteomalacia
Hemochromatosis

Mechanical derangements of the spine
Spondylolisthesis
Spinal stenosis
Vertebral compression fractures
Intervertebral disk herniations
Scheuermann's disease

Miscellaneous causes
Retroperitoneal diseases (vascular, malignancies)
Referred pain from abdominal or pelvic organ pathology
Abdominal aneurysm
Paget's disease of bone
Herpes Zoster

that has a wide expression in variance—dependent on gender, age, culture and even comorbid diseases, all of which affect our ability to tolerate and live with chronic pain.

Ultimately, the severity of pain may not be as important a marker as some of the other flags on the list. In any case, having a single Red Flag is certainly not reason to panic, but certain combinations of these flags should raise your index of suspicion. Unquestionably, the more flags present, the more likely that there is a significant problem that requires addressing.

Most important: pay attention to the internal barometers of changing health

If, for example, you have a previous history of cancer, osteoporosis, or have been using the drugs in question for some time and, in addition to your back pain, you develop new symptoms that you are unable to explain, you certainly have a very good reason to schedule a visit with your physician, without delay, to address these new developments.

Most important is the need to pay attention to the internal barometers of changing health. If we pay attention to our bodies, almost always we will be alerted to an adverse change in our general well being. The group of medical problems with back pain that we are discussing, will most likely not spontaneously improve or go away, and the course will almost always be characteristically marked by a progressive deterioration. We will feel generally unwell in addition to the back pain and, almost always, if we are conscientiously attentive to our health, we will have some sense that this is not an ordinary backache.

This deteriorating state of affairs should start the bells ringing and prompt the individual to consult their attending physician without procrastination, so that the underlying cause can be identified and

The 7 Red Flags of Back Pain

1. Loss of control of limbs, bladder or bowel

2. Night symptoms: sweats or significant pain that prevents sleep

3. Constitutional symptoms: fever, unexplained weight loss, gross fatigue

4. Prolonged use of specific drugs: steroids, immunosuppressive drugs, intravenous drugs

5. Previous history of cancer

6. History of significant fall or trauma—especially if associated with osteoporosis

7. Unexplained and increasing pain

managed appropriately. Experienced clinicians are aware that, in many cases, patients may have had the feeling that something was wrong for some time before presenting for medical help, fear often being the mitigating factor delaying presentation.

Remember, almost all of these problems can be treated successfully and, if not resolved with appropriate management, the course of the disease can be effectively managed to minimize any catastrophic outcome.

Sciatica and Other Spinal Nerve Compression Syndromes

There is one specific type of back pain that occurs commonly enough that it requires special attention and discussion. This type of back or neck pain is associated with pain radiating down an extremity, either an arm or leg, but far more commonly a leg. The cause of this radiating pain, regardless of whether it involves the upper or lower extremity, is similar and the medical management of these two scenarios is virtually identical.

When the pain radiates from the back or neck into one of the extremities, especially if it goes past the knee or elbow, it generally signifies that there is pressure on a spinal nerve, most commonly at its root soon after it branches off from the spinal cord and is exiting from the spinal column. When this phenomenon occurs in the lower extremity, it is commonly referred to as sciatica, an irritation of one or more of the spinal nerve roots comprising the sciatic nerve—the major nerve coursing down the leg, responsible for essentially all the neurological functions of that lower extremity.

Prolonged loss of nerve supply to the muscle will result in clinically measurable shrinkage of muscle mass

The cause of sciatica or any other nerve compression syndrome may vary from a minor irritation of the nerve caused by spasm of the muscles through which the nerve or its component nerve roots must pass, to a significant anatomical displacement of the nerve roots caused by a protruded or ruptured vertebral disc, osteophytic bone spur or—very uncommonly—a tumor mass.

In all cases, investigative tests will, in all probability, correctly identify what is causing the pressure on the nerve, and will indicate the need for either urgent surgical intervention or, more likely, the requirement of a conservative and supportive medical management program.

Nerves develop like co-axial cables with the sensory fibers being on the outside of the nerve and the inner fibers of the nerve comprising the motor fibers that provide the electrical signals to the contractile elements of muscle. Accordingly, with conditions that produce only small amounts of pressure on the nerve, the initial symptoms experienced will be pain and *paresthesia*, a medical term describing dysfunction of sensation experienced as numbness or tingling and indicating that the nerve dysfunction is confined to the sensory portion of the nerve.

> 80% of patients show improvement and recovery within a year— without the need for surgical intervention

With increasing anatomical pressure on the nerve and growing displacement of the inner motor fibers of the nerve supplying the intended distal muscles, the affected individual will begin to note changes in specific motor strength, with increasing weakness when compared to the same muscles on the unaffected limb.

This loss of nerve supply to the muscle will result not only in weakness of the affected limb, but, over time, eventual wasting and atrophy of the affected muscles, with a clinically measurable shrinking in circumference of the affected limb. The magnitude of motor loss in the clinical syndrome is almost always indicative of the severity of the problem, and is a reasonably good marker of the measure of convalescence necessary to return to normal status.

Treatment of these nerve compression syndromes is almost always addressed initially with a conservative management program combining any number of the physical therapies we have discussed earlier, along with the necessary prescribed pain management medications as required to ease the patient through the acute phase.

How Should Sciatica be Managed?

It is important to know that these compression nerve syndromes are hardly ever surgical emergencies, and invariably most specialists in the field would suggest a minimum of three months of rehabilitation therapy, in the absence of any ongoing deterioration, prior to consideration of surgical intervention.

Treated conservatively, the natural history of these radicular syndromes results in 80% of patients showing progressive improvement and recovery over the course of a year, without the need of any surgical intervention. The success of the medical management program is likely dependent on the correct mix of therapeutic modalities, as well as a proper exercise program to resolve problems relating to core strength and axial stability.

Failure to address this axial stability, which is likely an underlying and contributing cause of the original injury, may very well result in reoccurrence of the same syndrome within a short period of time. Even the most encouraging therapists sometimes find their previously enthusiastic patients less motivated to participate in their prescribed exercises, as their symptoms improve.

It is unfortunate that in many of these cases, relapse must occur before exercise programming is tackled with the conviction necessary to resolve the problem.

Unfortunately, in spite of everyone's best efforts, the other 20% of these nerve compression syndromes will decline further with increasing weakness and symptom deterioration, requiring surgical decompression to prevent further decompensation and degeneration of musculoskeletal function.

This need for surgery falls under two separate groups. The first group that we have just discussed describes an "absolute indication" and almost always involves a progressive neurological deficit of the affected limb. The implication is that the pressure on the nerve is increasing in spite of a "best efforts", conservative management therapy, resulting in a progressive loss of the function of the involved nerve in its role of enervating the limb. Surgical decompression is generally indicated to restore the function of the nerve and recovery of the muscle function.

The second category leading to surgical intervention is less common and refers to a "relative indication". In this group, although the muscular function of the limb is preserved, the pain continues unabated with significant deterioration in quality-of-life. In these cases, a clinical decision is made regarding the ability of the patient to tolerate the level of discomfort, and palliative surgical management may be offered to preserve quality-of-life and allow the individual to resume normal activity.

It is important for the attending surgeon in these cases to be confident, based on investigations undertaken, that surgical intervention will result in a significant and measurable improvement in the patient's presenting symptom complaint.

It is regrettably possible that the ill-fated individual may have the surgery but still find himself or herself only minimally improved postoperatively. This unfortunate group of "failed surgical backs", although hopefully representative of only a small fraction of the presenting group, will continue to suffer symptoms of back pain and pain radiation to the arm or leg.

Reading Notes:

PART II

THE 7 PROMISES OF PERFECT POSTURE

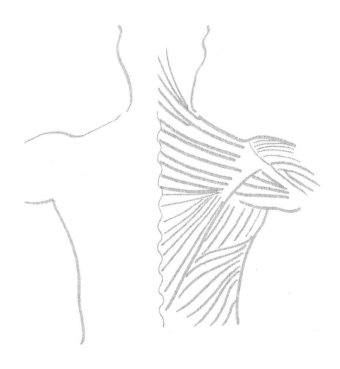

Promise #1:
Your Bones Will
Grow Stronger

U nderstanding the Difference: Osteopenia, Osteoporosis and Osteoarthritis

When it comes to bones, after the age of 30, everything is downhill all the way. By 30, both men and women will have reached their peak bone mass and, from this time forward, the only options available to us are to slow down the inevitable decline of age and use what bone producing (osteogenic) capabilities we have to maintain the very strongest skeleton possible.

This rate of progression in both men and women will be influenced by several factors; but, without fail, in all of us there will be a gradual deterioration and loss of bone density. Although more marked in women, this trend of deterioration will affect men as well.

On average, after age 30, women will lose approximately 1% of total bone density each year until the onset of menopause, at which time this rate will double or triple—sometimes with significantly harmful results.

This change in bone metabolism is defined by two terms: *osteopenia* and *osteoporosis*.

7 PROMISE

Osteopenia is a term indicating less than normal standards of bone density in our skeleton when compared to other individuals in our age peer group. This person with osteopenia cannot yet be described as having *osteoporosis*, which defines a more advanced loss of bone mass (defined statistically as greater than 2.5 standard deviations less than the majority of people who are their age) but they are well on their way.

Osteoporosis is, in essence, a silent disease

By the time you have osteoporosis, statistically there is a significant risk of fracture. The reason is simple enough. The loss of calcium over the intervening years has resulted in a weakening of the bony matrix to the point that, if subjected to a severe blow or fall it will likely result in a fracture.

To clarify, one should again mention *osteoarthritis*, which is often confused in the discussion of *osteoporosis* and *osteopenia*.

Osteoarthritis refers to the "wearing out" degenerative arthritis that affects all of us, should we be fortunate enough to live so long. Although osteoarthritis may coexist alongside *osteopenia* and *osteoporosis,* they are otherwise unrelated.

Osteopenia and *osteoporosis* are all about bone density, which is defined by the amount of calcium seeded throughout the matrix of bone giving it its strength.

Osteoporosis, osteopenia and *osteoarthritis,* however, do have one thing in common when it comes to backs: all three of them are generally without symptoms until something happens.

Osteoporosis, until it results in a fracture or collapse of bone matrix, is in essence a silent disease.

It generally comes as quite a surprise to most people when they find out that they have osteoporosis, often discovered after their doctor orders a routine screening bone density test when they enter middle age. It comes as even a greater surprise to find out that they have osteoporosis when they arrive in the emergency department after tripping and falling only to find out that they have a fractured wrist or hip and need to be in a cast for six weeks or, worse yet, in intensive rehabilitation for three months to recover from a fractured hip.

In most cases, the event causing the osteoporotic fracture will produce enough pain that it is likely the diagnosis will be made upon presentation to the emergency department.

In other cases, however, the collapse of bone may not be caused by a specific event, but will occur gradually over time and commonly be unassociated with any discomfort. In these cases, the vertebral bodies comprising the spinal column will be gradually crushed at the front, associated with a gradual deterioration in posture resulting in a bone deformity of the spine known as *kyphosis*. Kyphosis describes the development of the classical hunchback that can develop with age, also known as a "dowagers hump"—another unflattering term left over from the Victorian era describing an elderly widow of high social station.

There are a number of factors that may predispose us to developing osteoporosis more than other people. Some of these factors relate to lifestyle choices whereas others are just a matter of "luck of the draw".

Who your ancestors are may increase the risk of osteoporosis—with some races more at risk than others. If there is a family history of osteoporosis, especially in a close relative, the higher the risk. And, lastly, the earlier the onset of menopause if you are a woman, the more likely you will experience a faster decline in skeletal strength.

There are other risk factors related to lifestyle which also increase the risk of osteoporosis: smoking, excess use of alcohol and diets that are too low in calcium and vitamin D. Choices that favor physically sedentary lifestyles are also significant contributory factors that accelerate the onset of osteoporosis.

> **Choices that favor physically sedentary lifestyles accelerate the onset of osteoporosis**

All of these factors are associated with accelerated bone loss and the accompanying complications relating to osteoporosis.

Although we cannot choose our ancestors, it is satisfying to know that there are some choices that we can make to postpone the inevitable advance of age—at least as it relates to bone health. In fact, if we look around us, there are a fair number in their advanced years whose "bone skeletons" are still quite sprightly, a result of choices that they made as they progressed through the middle years.

The earlier we begin taking these measures, the more successful we are in maintaining our skeletal health. Rebuilding the matrix of osteoporotic bone after a spinal vertebral collapse or a fractured hip is a very slow process indeed.

The practice of minimizing lifestyle abuses for most of us is a "work in progress", with some periods of our life celebrating more success than others. A diet adequate in calcium and vitamin D is simple enough to acquire in industrialized countries, and should never be a reason for development of osteoporosis, which leaves us with interpreting what qualifies as a "physically sedentary lifestyle".

One thing of which science is sure: healthy bone—especially *axialskeletal bone*—must be subjected to stress or weight-bearing to achieve maximum health and strength. The term *axialskeletal* refers to those bony parts of us that support our total body weight when we are in the erect position.

The microscopic structure of bone matrix in axialskeletal bone is different, for example, from non-weight-bearing bone such as in our fingers or arm. Bones that are designed to bear weight, develop in a specialized way to withstand this stress of weight bearing, and are continually remodeled throughout life, dependent on the physical demands placed upon them. The "girders of calcium" that define this specialized bone matrix are preferentially laid down in a bioengineered matrix optimally designed to cope with the gravitational stress placed upon it.

This genetically evolved system that matches architectural bone mass and structure to functional demand is known in bone physiology as *functional adaptation*. This ability to preferentially strengthen different parts of our skeletons more than others, and continually adapt to the changing gravitational forces imposed on our skeleton as our posture changes with neglect or age, provides us with a safety valve keeping our fracture risk at an acceptable biological level.

Why Astronauts Get Osteoporosis

This entire process, however, is dependent on one thing: the bone must be subjected to a dynamic stress. The easiest way to study bone in the absence of any stress is to look at astronauts in space, in the absence of gravity, a condition results in what is referred to in bioengineering terms as *skeletal unloading*.

After only two weeks of enforced bed rest, bone building and re-modeling come to a complete standstill

The immediate consequence of skeletal unloading in space is a rapid reabsorption of calcium and development of bone loss. On earth, we also can find evidence of skeletal unloading where, in circumstances of enforced bed rest, after only two weeks, bone building and remodeling come to a complete standstill. Immediately, the reverse process begins and demonstrable changes of re-absorption of calcium can be measured as the deteriorating course of osteoporosis is activated.

Interestingly enough, very little effort is needed to change and reverse this deteriorating affect. While orbiting in space, merely having the astronauts provide a simple mechanical stimulus by tapping their heel bone against something firm several times a day, while they are going about their daily business, changed this calcium reabsorption process in the heel bone.

This straightforward action will provide sufficient enough dynamic strain along the weight-bearing axis of the foot, to arrest the bone resorption and enhance new bone formation, a change that is observable shortly after initiating the instruction to the astronauts. This uncomplicated effort is all that is necessary to trigger a measurable osteogenesis and formation of new bone in the heel.

How Chronic Back Pain Causes Osteoporosis

This is very good news for people who have chronic postural back pain for, unfortunately, they are a group of people who find themselves at risk of developing osteoporosis at much earlier ages than people who do not have this complaint. The reason is quite easily explained, because chronic back pain sufferers almost always have more sedentary lifestyles.

To diminish intensity of pain, chronic back pain sufferers characteristically reduce activity as their coping strategy. The increasingly sedentary way of life and inactivity comes with a cost, however, resulting in acceleration of resorption of calcium and an ever-decreasing bone mass. We have to reconsider this strategy if we want to reverse the process.

It may surprise you to find out that, much like the astronauts, we have to do very little to change this. Using the scientific advancements of *bioengineered loading phenomena* described earlier, to create new bone and give that bone optimal strength, all we have to do is subject that bone to a dynamic stress along the axial line most requiring the strength.

The osteoporosis studies conducted in space laboratories suggest that even holding correct postural stance for short periods of time during the course of the day will result in the provision of the necessary dynamic strain to the axialskeletal system along its proper axis, and increasing the bone strength along this very important axial line.

In other words, the simple act of maintaining perfect posture, resulting in the appropriate dynamic strain being applied to the precise axial gravitational line supporting our upright body, will

The simple act of maintaining perfect posture results in the maintenance of the optimal matrix of bone

have the consequence of the optimal matrix of bone being laid down, providing the maximal strength along the gravitational stress line of our weight-bearing skeleton.

There is a certain irony that maintaining perfect posture provides the single most preventative measure we can adopt in preventing the natural deterioration of bone reabsorption in our axialskeletal system and ensuring its optimal strength.

It is only a matter of time before the physician managing a patient with postural back pain and early osteoporosis will be faced with the inevitable question: "What exercise and how much is enough?"

Cutting to the chase, everyone wants to find out the bottom line as they begin implementing a daily program that they can live with. A minimal program that we can adhere to regularly is significantly better than any program that is doomed before it starts because we can't find the time to carry it out.

And what is the best answer to this question?

As much as possible during the course of the day, whether sitting or standing, make your very best efforts in maintaining ideal, perfect posture.

And...

Walk!

Walk every chance you get—even for short distances! Walk rather than ride whenever you can! Take the stairs!

Just walk!

> In the end, it is the choices we make and the actions we take

All the medical studies have suggested that this commitment to holding proper, erect posture combined with ordinary walking is the very best body training to resist the aging process of osteoporosis and create the anabolic stimulus needed for ideal bone regeneration and optimal skeletal strength.

In the end, it is the choices that we make and the actions we take, based on the exercise of our personal empowerment, that provide the only positive stimuli to effectively encourage preservation of healthy bone metabolism.

In doing this, we will ensure that our axialskeletal foundation is able to maintain its greatest strength in the force plane required to prevent a potential fracture from occurring because, for most of us, it is only a matter of time before we experience that inevitable tumble to the ground during a moment of distraction and inattention.

Promise #2: Your Back Muscles Will Heal with Greater Strength and Power

8

S trength and power are a function of muscular health. At first glance, it appears implausible to believe that merely maintaining proper posture can result in increased strength and power to core stabilizers; however, a quick primer on the pathophysiology of how injured muscle repairs and strengthens itself will quickly clarify the accuracy in this statement.

People who experience chronic postural back pain, will all exhibit pain with deep palpation of the structural paravertebral muscles in the involved spinal segments. This pain, which can involve one or more of the superficial, mid or deep layers of the supporting muscle, is evidence of inflammation and injury. In other words, if you are sore when you push, prod or poke it—the underlying muscle is injured and inflamed!

Moreover, the persistence of this chronic pain suggests that the injury is an ongoing phenomenon, coinciding with the simultaneous healing process of other parts of the same muscle.

The Unique Stages of Back Muscle Healing

Different body tissues heal and regenerate in different ways. When bone is injured, for example, the healing process is defined by a regenerative process, which produces a bone matrix that is virtually identical and indistinguishable from the previously injured bone. Healing of injured skeletal muscle, unlike bone, follows a different repair process. Following injury to the muscle, microscopic examination can clearly identify the morphological changes in the area of injury, including the extent and quality of the body's healing efforts.

Clinical research in the regenerative process clearly demonstrates that muscle healing can be affected by several factors over which we can exert control during the progressive phases of the repair process.

Examination of injured skeletal muscle demonstrates that the reparative process follows a consistent pattern, irrespective of the underlying cause of injury. The body makes no distinction between healing muscle fibers that have been violently torn during a motor vehicle accident or sporting injury, or the healing of a chronically strained muscle, such as we would see in chronic postural back pain syndromes.

> **Phagocytes arrive on the scene shortly after injury to mop up the cellular debris**

Each muscle is composed of many thousands of specialized muscle cells called *myofibrils*, bundled together with their respective nerve cells, connective tissue and blood vessels. It is these myofibrils that provide the contractile element characteristic of muscles. Myofibrils vary in length from a fraction of an inch as noted in the specialized muscles of hearing, controlling the minute auditory bones in the ear, to 24 inches long in the large running muscles of the leg. They can also vary in width from the thickness of a hair to over an inch in diameter in trained power lifters.

Interspersed throughout the population of these myofibrils in different muscle bundles, are satellite *stem cells*, embryonic leftovers, which will provide precursors to create the new populations of myofibrils we require to replace damaged muscle fibers from injuries experienced throughout our life.

The initial phase of repair following a muscle injury involves infiltration of *phagocytes*, specialized cells produced by the body, which arrive on the scene shortly after the injury to mop up the cellular debris produced by ruptured muscle cells. These phagocytes, working much like a colony of army ants picking clean a carcass laying on the forest floor, leave behind the old skeleton matrix on which the new myofibrils will be laid out and constructed.

After this initial cleanup, stem cells, the body's regenerative building blocks referred to earlier, are triggered into action in a complex biological process. Having lain dormant in the muscle from the time of fetal development, these and other stem cells from adjacent tissue, as well as those seeded into the area by infiltrating blood, begin development into new muscle cells, aligning themselves to the underlying matrix left behind by the phagocytes, to form the new contractile components in the regenerated muscle. At the same time, fibroblasts and other connective tissue cells lay down collagen fibers in the production of healing scar tissue, accompanied by the new ingrowth of capillary blood vessels to supply nutrients and oxygen for the newly developed muscle fibers.

The final remodelling phase is similar to a "work hardening program" whereby the repaired muscle, comprised of newly generated myofibrils, begins its new task, training and adapting to the stresses placed upon the muscle, undergoing reorganization until all the hardened contractile myofibrils are capable of providing the functional capacity required of that particular muscle group.

Whereas in an acute single injury, the phases of repair may be seen as separate, contiguous events starting from an initial injury and progressing to an end-stage healed muscle, in chronic back strain, we have an ongoing, overlapping of injury, healing and reinjury, with the various repair phases at different stages in the cycle of regeneration.

How to Accelerate the Muscle Healing Process in Chronic Back Pain

Of interest to clinicians is the timing and duration of these stages in healing, as well as the various factors and elements that influence the process. It has been demonstrated that this healing process can be influenced both in a supportive as well as an injurious manner.

Failure to introduce range-of-motion exercises will result in an inadequately repaired muscle and perpetuation of injury

During the very early stages of healing immediately following injury, there is strong evidence indicating that rest and immobilization, defined for a structured convalescent period, are critical to the healing process in the first four to seven days. Failure to respect this rule will result in both prolongation of the healing process, as well as a reduction in the eventual strength of the inadequately repaired muscle.

After this early period of immobilization, it is equally critical to introduce range of motion exercises within the physiological range of motion specific to that muscle, to ensure optimal healing. In fact, failure to provide this physiological range of motion, will not only delay the healing of the injured muscle, but will result in the regenerated muscle attaining only a portion of its prior original functional strength and extensibility, giving rise to the probability that the inadequately repaired muscle will experience reinjury and perpetuation of the injury cycle.

This ability for human muscle to regenerate from stem cells to mature myofibrils persists right into advanced old age. The number of stem cells is greatest immediately after birth, when they comprise 15% of the population of all muscle cells. This begins to fall off quickly thereafter and by the age of two, the levels have dropped to 10% and, by adulthood, number only 4%, drifting off progressively as we age.

This allows us to manage the healing of sprains and strains right into our *golden years* but the rate of healing is considerably slower than it was at age 21—a fact which most of us hardly need science to remind us! What is important to know, however, is that it is this regular performance of exercise that ensures optimal cellular maintenance of stem cells. Absence of exercise results in their premature demise, fulfilling the observed axiom: *Use it or lose it!*

Of importance, as well, is the role of scarring and fibrosis during the healing of injured muscle. From a functional standpoint, it is desirable to minimize scarring and fibrosis because scar displaces the available space for myofibrils in the muscle body, reducing the overall contractile function of that specific muscle.

Whereas it has been long thought that the scarring process was intrinsic and unchangeable in the healing process of muscle, recent research has suggested that scar tissue will develop preferentially in healing muscles forced into immobilization—especially if this immobilization is prolonged past the initial prescribed period of rest. The healthiest population of healed myofibrils, with the least amount of scarring, occurs in healing muscles that are subjected to regular and periodic physiologic range-of-motion exercises during the regenerative process.

Do Medicines and Supplements Play a Role in Muscle Healing?

As one might expect, there are a number of biological growth factors and inflammatory mediators that are involved in the healing of injured muscle tissue. Many of these biological activators have been studied for their affect on the muscle regenerative process, with the hopes of being able to positively enhance healing. Clinical studies, including direct injection of growth factors into healing muscle, however, to date have not demonstrated any evidence of beneficial effects.

Long-term use of anti-inflammatories may be detrimental to the healing of muscle tissue

Although it is exciting to speculate as to what role stem cell and gene therapy, growth factors or precursor supplements may have in future breakthroughs in the muscle healing process, there is little clinical evidence, at present, to suggest that use of these biological agents as supplements are useful in mediating this regenerative process. The scientific understanding, at present, is that this regenerative process involves the biological activity of these various growth factors in a complexly regulated expression, with specific actions exerted at precise times and at precise, specific sites. Until this spatial temporal cycle can be clearly understood, serious consideration of therapeutic use of these growth factors and other supplement precursors, at present, can only be considered speculative and poorly validated.

This can also be said for many of the physician-prescribed medicines used commonly today. Prescriptions or injections of glucocorticoids or steroids in the treatment of acute muscle injuries will delay the healing process and, unless there is some other compelling clinical reason for their use, the use of steroids should probably be restricted, as they would seem to interfere with the healing process of muscle tissue itself.

Nonsteroidal anti-inflammatories (NSAIDs), although perhaps somewhat beneficial in terms of symptom relief in the recovery from exercise-induced strain, also do not appear to contribute to healing, either in accelerating the healing process or improving the eventual outcome. Long-term use of NSAIDs, in fact, may be detrimental to the healing of muscle tissue. In some studies of the eccentric contraction-induced strain injury model, progress in healing was actually inhibited by their use.

The conclusion of current research supports the premise that the only effective method of assisting healing of an injured muscle is to subject the recovering injured muscle to a structured, physiological range-of-motion exercise program, ensuring adequate stretching and controlled dynamic stress stimulation on a regular treatment schedule. This will result in the injured muscle bundle being colonized with the healthiest population of myofibrils, with the least amount of scar tissue and the repaired muscle fibers optimally hardened to perform the task required of that specialized muscle group.

This also explains why chronic back pain sufferers have weak backs. Clinical studies have repeatedly demonstrated that patients experiencing chronic back pain consistently and almost continually restrict moving the vertebral segments that give them pain.

This would seem a most natural response because of the associated pain increase that accompanies physical activity. The decreased level of activity unfortunately contributes to further wasting of trunk musculature, a decrease in muscular strength and endurance, muscle spasms, stiffness of ligaments and joints, and reduced metabolic activity, all deleterious effects provoked by disuse. This results in a perpetual deconditioning syndrome, a defining characteristic of people with chronic postural back pain.

> A good understanding of core stabilization is very useful to the person with chronic postural backache

Laboratory examination of patients with chronic back pain, using real-time ultrasound examination and electromyographic studies studying muscle electrical activity with fine wire insertion and surface electrodes, confirms this evidence.

All of these patients demonstrate evidence of dysfunctional motor control as well as atrophy and power loss in both local and global muscle core stabilizers where strength may only approach 70% of normal expected levels.

The Role of Core Stabilization in Healing Chronic Back Pain

A key buzzword in the lucrative exercise business today is *core stabilization*. Many people have a vague idea of this concept but a good understanding of the doctrine of core stabilization is very useful to the person with chronic postural backache because it helps them understand what they must do differently to produce a change in their back pain.

The core stability concept is not difficult to understand. The spinal column, which represents the foundation to our posture, can be compared to a mast of a sailing ship, where the strength and stability of the mast is dependent on the "shrouds and stays" that support it from different angles anchored to the ship's deck and hull. Although the spinal column is dynamically mobile, the analogy of support is nevertheless valid, with different groups of muscles surrounding the spine, acting like the shrouds and stays, each having a specific function and responsibility in support of the functional upright spine.

There are three different groups of muscles, which individually number into the hundreds, working independently, as well as together in concerted team efforts, providing this postural stabilization.

The first level of core strength muscles are identified as *local stabilizers*, whose function is to provide individual vertebral segmental stability. Responsible only for controlling stability in relationship to its nearest neighbouring vertebral body, they have no role in production of movement. These muscles work continuously, as long as we are upright, as opposed to muscles designed to produce movement, which need often be active only during the actual movement itself.

Surprisingly enough, in spite of the tremendous work expected of them, the vast majority of these first-level muscles are no bigger than the length or thickness of the little finger on your hand; yet, it is the orchestrated effort of these small muscles that provides for the overall stability of the spinal column.

The second level of muscles called *global stabilizers*, work over several vertebral segments, generating stability and force. They bridge the span of a greater number of vertebral bodies, controlling the complex range of spinal movements including flexion, extension, side bending and torsion. As noted earlier, the activity of these muscles is noncontinuous, with the electrical firing only apparent when the intended movement is executed, facilitating an overall coordination and stability of the vertebral column.

The third and last group of muscles are considered *global mobilizers*. These muscles are less involved in stabilization, but provide the muscular strength in producing the effort required for energy-expending tasks. The activities of these muscles, like the global stabilizers, are again noncontinuous and demonstrate activity only during periods of required effort. They are, however, immediately recruited for stability when we place our spine under a load, such as with a heavy lift, or performance of a quick ballistic movement, as in lunging to catch a vase tipping off a nearby counter.

The weakness in chronic postural backache sufferers has been specifically identified to be the small multifidis muscles, the very same little-finger-thickness, first-level inner-core small muscles previously mentioned, bridging each vertebral body to its adjacent neighbors, providing the necessary vertical stability along the centered gravitational axis.

For this reason, core stabilization exercise programs are structurally designed to address this weakness. The most sophisticated exercise programs use exercise therapists who are aided with real-time ultrasound equipment. Using the benefit of biofeedback experience helps isolate the recognition of movement in these very small and specialized muscles. Because the mass of these muscles are so small in comparison to the other prime movers of the spine, it is often very difficult to recognize their specific contribution.

In those subjects whom benefit from this guided exercise programming, it is difficult, however, to isolate the perceived, added benefit of the improved learning curve provided by this sophisticated tool and its contribution to the overall treatment management of chronic postural back pain. In any case, because of the relative unavailability of this treatment program, it is perhaps more useful to find an alternate path to achieve this desired result, one not requiring the need of a sophisticated laboratory.

> A focused effort at maintaining balanced postural positioning results in the ideal exercise program

We know from numerous muscle physiology studies that, in order to maintain a stable, balanced posture, each of these small, intrinsic multifidus muscles must be optimally working and firing to provide a centered and balanced gravitational vertical axis.

Therefore, a focused effort at maintaining this balanced postural position results in the ideal exercise program, providing an optimal strengthening and hardening workout for the maturing myofibrils, essentially asking the developing myofibrils to do the exact work expected in their predestined task of maintaining perfect posture.

This simple act of maintaining proper posture will result in the ideal exercise routine. Adding a progressive strengthening training program with resistant exercises will add further, significant increments in the restoration of the muscles bulk and strength.

How to Schedule an Exercise Recovery Program

First efforts at maintaining perfect posture often result in development of stiffness in various muscle groups and raised eyebrows questioning the wisdom of pursuing the new postural stance. The initial effort to pull the body into normal postural alignment is counteracted by an uncomfortable awareness of muscle tightening in a quickly identified group of opposing muscles, preventing the easy transition back into neutral plane alignment.

> The initial effort to pull the body into normal postural alignment is counteracted by uncomfortable muscle tightening

This muscular restriction will be felt in the *prime movers* of that person's dominant activities where the muscle has undergone a relative hypertrophy or over-development, while the opposing muscle groups are characterized by a relative weakness. This is quite easily demonstrated in most people when it comes to the strong pectoralis muscles in the upper chest—muscles that we continually exercise all day long by pushing, pulling, and lifting.

Almost always, these stronger muscles will overpower the shoulder-girdle and pull the shoulders forward, feeling uncomfortably tugged on when we try to stand or sit up straight by pulling the shoulders backward. The muscular effort of the relatively underdeveloped and weakened scapular muscles between the shoulder blades—trying to pull the "wing bones" backwards into a normal postural stance—are easily overcome by the overdeveloped chest muscles.

This common muscle imbalance creates the typical picture identified with poor shoulder girdle posture, producing the fatigued and forward hunched shoulders that describes many of us at the end of a tiring day.

The quickest way to improve this picture is not to focus on a strengthening program but rather to make a concentrated effort on improving the flexibility and give of the overtightened chest muscles with an effective stretching program. This itself will provide an immediate improvement in comfort by allowing us to straighten and lift our shoulders, approaching neutral plane alignment.

> Only after an effective stretching program should efforts be directed to strengthening

Only after ensuring that muscles have been adequately worked out with an effective stretching program, should efforts be directed to the strengthening process.

Almost everyone who eventually sees the light and begins an effective exercise program, even after ample warning, will overdo the muscular effort with start-up of an exercise program, in the misguided effort to catch up on lost time. This will inevitably result in an inflammation flare-up, causing an increased level of discomfort.

The old weight-lifting advice of going at it until you can feel the strain does not apply in this case and, in fact, will set you back as your body once more goes through the cycle of inflammatory flare-up and healing.

A good rule of thumb is to start with your exercise program at a point you absolutely know will cause no difficulty and then increase the program by 10% every third workout, either in effort *or* repetitions of movement—***but not both***. This will allow your body plenty of time to adapt to any changes and demands placed upon it, without the risk of adding further strain.

Finding that centered vertical axis of positioning that is neutral for your body *today*, is what you must seek. The effort you will have to expend to maintain correct posture will vary throughout the day. It is generally difficult to adopt a good postural stance first thing in the morning after awakening, but after limbering up and stretching, we generally find our most balanced postural stance and available energy in the early part of the day. As the evening approaches, the onset of fatigue may contribute to more difficulty maintaining this correct posture.

The kinaesthetic appreciation of perfect posture is recognized when the naturally stronger muscles are relaxed and supple while the counteracting balancing muscles, which have a basic tendency to be ineffectually passive, are attentively contributing their balanced input towards the attainment of neutral plane posture.

Maintaining neutral plane alignment is a win-win situation!

Using personal empowerment to consciously put into practice the efforts required to attain perfect postural alignment will result in strengthening of the very muscles required to maintain this ideal alignment.

The 7 Promises of Perfect Posture

Reading Notes:

Promise #3: Your Back Pain Will Get A Lot Better

I t is not surprising to find out that pain is the most common symptom for which people seek medical attention. Each year 15% to 20% of us will present for treatment of pain resulting from an acute injury, and up to 30% of us will suffer chronic pain from which we can get little relief.

Chronic postural back pain sufferers form a large percentage of that chronic pain group.

How Feeling Pain Differs from Person To Person

How we neurologically process pain and the level to which each of us experience pain is widely variable. Given identical conditions and manifestations of the same disease, you will find one individual continuing to live a full, productive life but, on questioning, will admit to the presence of an uncomfortable, nagging pain. Another individual with the identical problem will find himself or herself confined to house and home, completely disabled with their affliction.

This dichotomy of pain response can produce problems for both patient and caregiver alike. Whereas the patient often feels an underlying lack of empathy to the amount of pain that they are feeling and the affect it is having on their life, an inexperienced therapist or even family member may have the

9 PROMISE

93

impression that the patient is indulging in their disability rather than getting on with their life.

The answer to the question, of course, is that pain is processed differently by different people. Pain tolerance cannot be confined to physiological explanation because it can be widely affected by a number of variables, which affect the individual's ability to be neurologically distracted by a higher order of priority. These neural rearrangements that define the *"organizational right of way"* through the processing of information by higher brain centers and the bringing of it to the conscious level, are vastly different from person to person.

Dramatic examples of these neurosensory priorities make interesting news stories with reports of individuals experiencing catastrophic injuries and still being able to overcome their pain, performing miraculous deeds in the process of saving themselves or others.

Less theatrical but equally heroic is the example of the mother with a chronic pain disability who gets up every morning before her family arises, taking care of all the chores required to see her children off to school competently and without fanfare, and then setting off to perform a full day's work.

> Pain following an acute injury forces us to rest, allowing the reparative process to begin

Both of these individuals are able to create a paradigm shift in their central nervous system processors, adjusting the sensory appreciation of pain and its consequent impact on their life.

Clinical medicine does not have all the answers to explain these widely variable expressions and responses to pain, but in the last several decades, significant advances in neuroscience have provided insights into pain mechanisms that allow for a more rational understanding and approach to pain management.

The 2 Types of Pain and How to Tell Them Apart

Pain is not always a bad thing. As an anciently evolved physiological response, pain allows us to immediately react to danger such as when we touch a hot stove. Pain following an acute injury also forces us to rest, an adaptive behavior as we learned earlier, allowing the reparative process to begin and enforcing the necessary period of immobilization.

We can, therefore, describe pain as either an *adaptive* pain in which the process serves some function, or a *maladaptive* pain in which the pain itself becomes the malady.

We can also divide pain into two other categories: *nociceptive* and *neuropathic* pain. Nociceptive pain, taken from the root word *noxious,* implies exactly that—pain caused by a noxious stimulus. Neuropathic pain, on the other hand, is an example of a maladaptive pain and comes about as a result of damage to the nerves themselves.

As an essential, protective mechanism, nociceptive pain is the pain that we were talking about when touching a hot stove, alerting us that continuing contact with the hot stove will cause tissue damage. It is the type of pain that answers the question, "Does it hurt when I press here?" The neural pathways mediating nociceptive pain have been well documented in neuro-scientific studies and are well understood.

The process involves the conversion of any intense mechanical stimulus such as heat or a pinprick, into electrical signals by highly specialized nerve endings, which are then transferred along nerve pathways from the periphery to the central nervous system (CNS), where these signals are processed and acted upon.

Any time we poke or prod something that is painful, we are eliciting this nociceptive pain signal. Nociceptive pain that goes away with healing of an acute injury, such as with a cut or bruise, is relatively straightforward. Nociceptive pain that is ongoing, as in the example of chronic postural back pain, is more complicated.

Persistence of muscle spasm and the resultant inflammatory process characteristic of chronic postural back pain, results in a classical inflammatory, histological response. With muscle tissue injury and inflammation, significant changes occur at the cellular environment of the nerve endings, secondary to the influx of various inflammatory chemical mediators from the site of injury. These chemical mediators, leaking through the cell walls of the overworked and damaged muscle cells, cause a complex biochemical cascade phenomena resulting in the production of prostaglandins and protein kinases, biologically active molecules that act on the resident nerve endings, lowering their threshold of activation and essentially allowing them to fire indiscriminately upon minimal stimulation.

In the case of chronic back pain, this means that the physical demands of certain tasks and other stimuli that would normally not cause pain, now become responsible for a continuing threshold of pain, which filters into our conscious awareness. This ability for nerve endings to become overexcited in response to persistent nociceptive stimuli is called *peripheral sensitization.*

This peripheral sensitization triggers a second event in which the barrage of indiscriminate firing by the peripheral nerves results in the higher neurological centers in the spinal cord and the brain itself to become overly reactive with resultant inappropriate responses. This secondary inappropriate neurobiological response phenomena is called *central sensitization* and further contributes to the intensity and severity of the pain.

The end result is a shift in pain threshold, increasing the modulation of pain awareness, creating a throbbing problem where previously the same stimulus was a benign non-event.

If this doesn't sound bad enough, it can get a lot worse! At the very end of this pain scale, this maladaptive change will generate spontaneous and exaggerated pain with no apparent protective or reparative role, producing excruciating pain by mere gentle stroking of the hairs that grow on the skin overlying the affected painful area.

This new type of pain in its full-blown state is called *neuropathic pain* and represents an out-of-control expression of the pathological operation of the nervous system. Neuropathic pain signifies severe damage to the nervous system in its function relating to interpretation of pain stimuli.

Fortunately, in postural back pain the damage to the nervous tissue is hardly ever severe enough to produce neuropathic pain syndromes, but the inflammatory contribution to peripheral and central sensitization described earlier by the injured muscle tissue is in itself a very real phenomenon. Depending on the amount of accumulated damage present in the supporting musculature, the result can be a significant amount of pain that clearly makes us "sit up and take notice". Neuropathic pain, however, can result from sciatica and the other nerve compression syndromes discussed earlier in the section *The 7 Red Flags of Back Pain* and, in fact, comprise a significant percentage of the neuropathic pain syndrome group.

Why Improving Posture Makes Back Pain Better

There are a number of pharmacological agents that are used in treatment of pain syndromes, which we have discussed earlier. Fortunately, for most of us experiencing chronic postural back pain, there are a number of steps that we can take first to change the circumstances causing our pain before we find it necessary to commit ourselves to the regular use of pain killers to cope with the daily activities of living.

The obvious solution is to arrest the ongoing muscle injury. The muscle injury is essentially an ongoing overuse injury inflicted on the spinal muscles as they attempt to support the body against forces of gravity in the inappropriate and maladaptive ergonomic position in which we have put ourselves.

The damaged muscle fibers contributing to this inflammatory process may be the result of an acute injury. More likely, however, they are groups of myofibrils experiencing a premature demise, overtaxed and overburdened, expended like front-line soldiers in a poorly thought-out skirmish. It is these damaged muscle cells that become the source of the blameworthy inflammatory mediators, seeping through the damaged cell walls into the surrounding tissue space.

Working toward ideal posture balances muscular workload and arrests chronic pain patterns

Treating the resultant pain with pharmacological agents, blocking neural pathways of conscious awareness, is one option of management, but other steps are open to us as well. We can take steps to arrest the cause responsible for creating the damage.

Short of confining ourselves to bed, precluding the necessity of use of muscular effort to hold us in a upright stance, the next best solution is maintaining the erect body in a postural stance least likely to induce strain on the supporting spinal musculature.

Working towards attainment of ideal posture balances muscular workload and arrests the chronic strain patterns imposed on these overworked core muscles. In the end, it is our choices and the exercise of our personal empowerment that will prevent the very exaggerated pain responses created by peripheral and central nervous sensitization of chronically inflamed neuromuscular structures.

The choices we make, exercising our personal empowerment in the progressive journey towards ideal perfect posture, arrests the chronic strain on the supporting muscles. This simple accomplishment will stop the entire cascade phenomena responsible for the muscle injury and subsequent chemical mediator leakage. It is those choices that will prevent the peripheral and central nervous sensitization that results in the exaggerated pain responses produced by chronically inflamed neuromuscular structures.

Reading Notes:

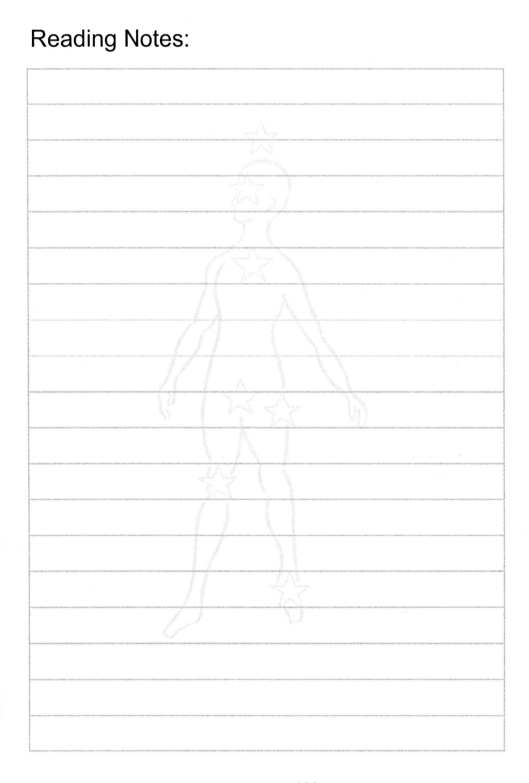

Promise #4:
Your Sense of Balance and Physical Poise Will Develop to a New Level

10

It is not difficult to agree upon the paramount, distinguishing characteristic associated with athleticism and youth. One needs to look no further than any exuberant group of neighborhood children milling about in play. Every playground activity associated with children—running, jumping, and skipping about with complete abandon and absence of fear, romping with an unreserved confidence in their physical prowess—points to postural balance as being the most decisive dynamic tying together the agility of youth.

Watching children acquire balance is probably one of the most fascinating activities that parents amuse themselves with during the early growing years of their infants and toddlers. Although not as quickly off the mark as a newborn antelope challenged with survival following birth, the toddler, following a brief neurological maturing process, soon enough becomes a handful for both parents. This learning curve characterizes the early developmental years as the child quickly grows and challenges the natural physiological boundaries that constrain the human form.

Understanding How Balance Works

The physiology of balance is a remarkable display of the rapid ability of the central nervous system to assimilate and act upon the multivariate information supplied by peripheral sensors distributed throughout the body, specializing in sensing many different types of information and numbered in the trillions. The central nervous system assembles this neurological data into a meaningful appreciation of the environment around the body, including the position that the body itself occupies relative to space and time. Having received this information, the brain then instantaneously and continuously sends back new commands to the body, altering its physical pose in response to a physiological demand to maintain an upright neutral-plane alignment, while the body constantly changes the dynamic *gravitational line of axis* as we move from one step to another.

To review our earlier discussion, this *gravitational axis line* describes an imaginary vertical line running upright through the erect body, through which the weight of the body torso, including the head and neck, is balanced both in front and behind, as well as from one side to the other. To maintain this gravitational axis line requires surprisingly little strength, especially when one pays attention to the awareness and maintenance of the body's center of balance.

The multiple and diverse neurological sensory centers maintaining this gravitational axis line are capable of input of the most innate minutia of data, all of which falls immeasurably below our level of consciousness—everything from the lightest feathery touch to our skin, to knowledge of the position of each weight-bearing joint of the body evaluating the stress upon it and comprehending the exact centeredness of the weight that each joint is distributing.

How Do We Control Balance?

Evaluation of the physiological controls of balance is exceedingly difficult for researchers to study because several groups of diverse proprioceptors provide input to maintain normal balance. Proprioceptors are those specialized neurological receptors whose sole purpose is to sense the position, orientation, location and movement of the entire body and its parts, continually streaming back information to the central nervous system. These proprioceptive sensors exist in every muscle, tendon and joint giving steady and continuous feedback to the brain.

When we think of disorders of balance that cause disability, it is common for us to automatically focus on the inner ear, located deep in our skull bones, which undoubtedly is the most singularly crucial organ in our body that controls balance and often can go out of whack temporarily, even with the common cold. The inner ear organs responsible for balance control consist of two parts: the labyrinth and otolithic organs.

The labyrinth, looking similar to a snail shell, is composed of three semicircular canals embedded in our skull, which are filled with a fluid that moves as we move, signaling the brain as to the position of the body in space, detecting both its speed as well as any accompaniment of rotational head movement. The otolithic organs, comprised of the utricle and saccule, detect linear movement as we move through space. In addition, small calcium carbonate stones called otoconia are located in these organs, which displace when we move our heads up and down as in nodding, giving additional information to the brain and signaling our head position.

All three of these inner ear organs contain tiny hair cells that constantly monitor physical displacement of the microscopic fibers that accompany head movement. It is difficult to imagine how complex the brain's "interpretive live streaming" must really be.

There are also some very basic neurological reflexes that assist us in keeping the upright position that we have inherited phyllogenetically in our evolutionary track through time. These basic neurological, instinctive reflexes date back to our reptilian existence and describe reactive gross motor movements over which we have no appreciable control.

Two of these reflexes are the *posture stabilization vestibulo-spinal reflex* and the *gaze stabilization vestibulo-ocular reflex.* These reflexes, although not quite developed in humans to the degree of our pet felines, are the ones that we observe as a cat twists unerringly in the air when dropped upside down, landing gracefully on its feet. Another instinctive reflex describes the quick movements we make to recapture balance when thrown off by a step on a slippery floor, or lively changes in balance we make to avoid an ankle twist while walking on an uneven trail.

Balance, Ballerinas and Aging
—-It's Not Always What It Seems!

Age in itself does not compromise balance. Balance control is affected neither by gender nor age, a finding quite remarkable, as it was once commonly thought that balance would automatically deteriorate with advancing age. In the absence of obvious musculoskeletal or neurovascular problems, however, this does not appear to be the case. Testing has demonstrated that healthy seniors have equal balance capabilities when compared to their junior test subjects.

> Testing show that healthy seniors have balance capabilities equal to their junior counterparts

A number of different scientific tools have been developed to quantitatively evaluate balance control. Sensory organization tests, as well as other functional tests called *posturography studies,* have been designed to evaluate the different characteristics associated with balance control. Although most are capable of only limited diagnostic capabilities, the study tools have, however, given us a much clearer understanding of balance control and have helped dispel several speculative assumptions.

One such assumption related to age was noted earlier. Another assumption was that certain types of athletes might demonstrate better balance control than others. One might think, for example, that competitive gymnasts or dancers might have better balance control them amateur joggers.

Studies, in fact, have demonstrated that in testing balance control of athletes from various sports including soccer, handball, basketball, badminton, tennis, competitive gymnastics, swimming and jogging, only one group of athletes showed any significant dominance over the other groups in a "one leg standing balance" sports medicine study. This study, unexpectedly, showed basketball players as the only group of athletes able to stand out when it came to maintaining balance while perched on one leg.

So, what are the greatest challenges to balance? In studies of healthy people, researchers challenged subjects by standing them on a platform, which was rigged to incorporate mild swaying and tilting while the person was standing upon it. Of all the various somatosensory proprioceptive disturbances, closing the eyes and blocking out any visual clues had the most affect in disturbing control of balance.

Not surprisingly, the second most effective way was by disturbing the sensory information from "the root" by applying a vibrating device to the Achilles tendon and disturbing the sensory feedback from the planted foot. Applying the vibrating device to the Achilles tendon has no effect on strength or the ability of the calf muscle to contract, but confuses and masks the proprioceptive information that the foot is trying to send back to the brain. By degrading the stream of proprioceptive information from the foot to the brain, regarding the surface on which we are standing, we significantly compromise our ability to maintain balance.

Many different diseases, any of which can change the "playing field" when it comes to managing our balance, will affect these proprioceptive sensors. Both diseases affecting the peripheral nerves, called *peripheral neuropathies,* and chronic degenerative changes affecting the muscles, tendons, bones or joints, can interfere in the ability of these proprioceptors to function normally. These changes are likely to occur with the onset of any chronic inflammatory conditions such as arthritis or diabetes and may even occur as side effects of medications used to treat these chronic conditions.

> In the US, 90 million people (42% of the population) will seek medical attention for balance problems

With so many different organ systems necessary to input the diverse information required to maintain balance, it is not surprising to find, as reported in National Institute of Health statistics, that in the United States alone, as many as 90 million people or 42% of the population will experience balance problems requiring visits to their health practitioners. These occurrences tend to increase with age as more degenerative conditions accumulate and become one of the most common reasons why patients over the age of 75 visit a physician.

In the situation where diseases have compromised our balance, the ability to maintain upright stature becomes significantly affected even for the simplest of movements. Those unfortunates so afflicted will almost always require aids such as canes and walkers to ensure stability and prevent falls or injury. The worst affected will find themselves confined to wheelchairs.

With a Little Effort Balance Can Be Improved at Any Age

Even with disabled neurological and musculoskeletal systems, balance can almost always be improved and significantly honed at any age. Improving balance for any individual is essentially a return on investment relating to the amount of effort dedicated each day to maintain postural centeredness. This is achieved by working towards attainment of a balanced gravitational axis line of perfect posture—a position that our body is naturally seeking in any case to reduce the amount of energy it must expend in maintaining upright stature.

In reality, any effort directed towards improving posture results in improved balance. A significant body of physiological and medical research has been directed at examination of the relationship between balance and posture. Studies involving Taijiquan are probably the most numerous in this cohort of research.

> **Any effort directed at improving posture results in improved balance**

Taijiquan, or Tai Chi as it is sometimes called, is an ancient Chinese "balance" exercise practice that starts with a resting *homebase,* stable postural position and involves slow, purposeful, circular movements of the upper extremities, accompanied by planned, measured and stable steps in a prescribed form towards the four directions of a compass. These movements are all directed from the *homebase* and eventually return to the same initial *homebase* position of rest. Each step of this choreographed form is unhurriedly performed having first established a solidly planted foot. Slowly and deliberately, the body weight is transferred to the other foot, which is carefully placed in the direction of the intended movement.

An objective observer with a background in kinesiology, unfamiliar with the artful movement of Taijiquan, might describe what they were seeing as a rhythmic and methodical process of putting each joint in the body through its full, normal physiological range of motion while standing in a stable erect postural stance. And, in fact, this would be a very apt description of what is happening during the supple movements prescribed by the Taijiquan form.

Historically derived from training sessions of martial artists dating back to early Chinese civilization, each Taijiquan individual movement is either a prescribed defensive or offensive maneuver, as would be practiced by a foot soldier in the process of training for hand-to-hand combat. Through the ages, the movements, although retaining their basic form, have become more stylized and, in fact, today, few practitioners of Taijiquan train for the purpose of competing in full-contact combat. These surviving gentle moves of the form, however, do have the very important function, as noted earlier, of ensuring that each joint of the body, both weight-bearing and non-weight-bearing, is moved through its full physiological range of motion.

> Adherence to the ideal postural pose is the most striking feature of Taijiquan

What this same observer might also note is that throughout the Taijiquan form, meticulous attention is being paid to maintain perfect upright posture to ensure that the transfer of weight to each new step was carried out ensuring a balanced and graceful transfer of weight so that at no point in time is there any evidence of "falling" into the new pose.

The basic postural stance of Taijiquan is universally practiced by all martial artists to ensure a stable and firmly rooted pose. This commonly shared postural root provides an exquisite balance capable of providing resistance to, surprisingly, even the greatest of efforts to disturb its centered axial line of gravity, while capable at the same time of engendering an almost reflexive, lightning movement of outpouring energy.

Documentary texts and reports even of recent times describe Taijiquan Masters capable of profound rootedness with astonishing, published descriptions of their feet creating furrows on paths as they walked and a capability of fracturing tile when walking across courtyards.

The attention to posture is the basic denominator that links the many diverse martial Taijiquan forms, which literally number in the hundreds, each with subtle variations. Although distinguished by its own prescribed sequence of slow arm movements and various stepping patterns, all are performed in a measured and unhurriedly purposeful manner. In the end, it is the commonality of the balanced postural stance that permits the smooth and graceful transitional changes of body weight between weighted and unweighted leg, highlighting the "signature postural pose" recognized universally in Taijiquan.

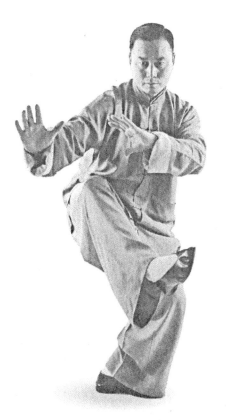

Although from the traditional Chinese medicine point of view, there may be a lot more than meets the eye in terms of the prescribed body movements of each form. From the Western medical point of view, it is the adherence to the ideal postural pose that is the most striking feature of the entire Taijiquan form.

With the reported health benefits documented in the public press over the course of the last several decades, the Western scientific and medical community has initiated and com-

Tung Hu Ling ...Tame the Tiger
reprinted with permission, Alex Dong, New York

pleted a significant block of studies to examine various aspects of improved health, reportedly generated from practicing Taijiquan; published studies that number in the thousands.

In statistical evidential terms, these research claims come forward in conclusions derived from meta-analytical studies. Meta-analytical studies involve researchers reviewing a large number of already completed studies, essentially a global examination of the entire archive of similarly published studies, focusing on a specific area of interest.

Each individual research study reviewed is graded in terms of its objectiveness in examining the specific area of focus. By reviewing large numbers of studies, the purpose of the meta-analytical study is to iron out statistical anomalies, thereby allowing the researchers to arrive at conclusions. These conclusions suggest a consensus of the evidence reported by the entire group of reviewed studies, all of which will have been undertaken by a diverse group of researchers, generally international in scope.

Considerable evidence suggests promising benefits from the regular practice of Taijiquan

In the end, these meta-analytical studies can give us a fairly accurate picture of general trends and a consensus of opinion in the specific area of focus. Taijiquan has been fortunate enough to benefit from several of these global studies.

In almost all of these studies, there was evidence that regular practice of Taijiquan resulted in demonstrable improvement in flexibility and dynamic balance control as well as enhancement of proprioceptive kinesthetic sensitivity and muscular strength. In terms of evaluating daily used physical activities, Taijiquan participants demonstrated measurable improvement in testing of both walking and running skills.

These improvements were noted even in patients who had previously been diagnosed with disabling conditions. Following the regular practice of Taijiquan, patients with dizziness and other central nervous system balance disorders demonstrated improvement both in postural control as well as in the ability to cope with imbalance. Patients with compromised motor skills resulting from multiple sclerosis also demonstrated improvements in walking speed by 21% after participation in Taijiquan training. With intensive therapy after even severe traumatic brain injury, there were significant improvements in walking skills following two to four years of Taijiquan training.

Although some of the studies measure the results of participants in Taijiquan over a period of months to years of practice, surprisingly, many of these enhanced health benefits were demonstrated in novice recruits who had been only recently introduced to Taijiquan with results measured after relatively short periods of participation.

One might also expect that these recruits were regular performers of the Taijiquan form, but, in fact, review of participation suggested quite the contrary. For example, one researcher noted that a 72% attendance at group class was described as "moderately good" and most participants in the study reported that their home practice sessions were, at best, "infrequent and inconsistent".

The common denominator to receiving all of these benefits appears to be very little else other than a concerted effort by individual study subjects to maintain a balanced effective posture, at least for the period of time each day supposedly dedicated to the practice of the Taijiquan exercise form. The in-

Patients with multiple sclerosis demonstrated a 21% improvement in walking speed after Taijiquan training

terpretation of these results suggests that the improved health parameters come as a result of *substantivity*, a term used to describe a sustained benefit that lasts following a previous treatment application. This appears to be a remarkable achievement in light of the less-than-enthusiastic and inconsistent participation in the daily practice of Taijiquan, with practice sessions lasting fewer than 30 minutes.

111

From the growing body of accumulated studies, one cannot over emphasize the significant physical benefits that result from the maintenance of a balanced postural stance. A compromise in balance at any age creates a significant disability. Even walking over uneven ground or traveling in a moving subway car can be a significant challenge to face if we do not have our balance.

> One cannot over emphasize the significant physical benefits that result from a balanced postural stance

On the other hand, if we dedicate time to paying attention and maintaining ideal posture, we become responsible for enhancing our personal empowerment and balance, ensuring increased personal freedom to explore the full scope of life that surrounds us.

Promise #5:
You Will Reduce Daily Stress Levels and Enhance Your Body's Biological Control Systems

11

C hronic pain syndromes are significant contributors to chronic stress disorders, a fact to which any physician in clinical practice can attest. The impact of stress caused by chronic back pain, like most biological conditions, can be graphically expressed by the classical *bell shaped curve* in affected populations. While at each end of this *bell shaped curve* there is a small group of people that either react very poorly or deal very effectively with stress, the great majority of us fill the large group in the center, coping with stress on a daily basis— sometimes successfully and other times poorly.

Many of the reasons why chronic back pain creates stress will be obvious. Certainly, the aggravating necessity to adapt our physical efforts and activities of daily living to our capabilities are obvious causes of mental stress, as we worry about meeting our own needs and those that depend on us. The presence of chronic pain induces fear, recognition that we may not have full control of our life. The fear of "loss of health" is one of the most deeply felt fears, causing physical and emotional stress. For some people, this fear is greater than the fear of death itself; for death is an endpoint, whereas chronic disability resulting in a painfully long life, is an even more bitter pill to swallow.

The Other Nervous System:
Autonomic Nervous System (ANS)

The presence of chronic worry creates changes in an entirely different biological arena, a playing field that exists below our level of awareness and control, and yet has very significant effects on our health and well being. This new arena where the battle with stress is fought, is our internal cellular environment, directed and moderated by our *autonomic nervous system (ANS)*.

When most people think of the nervous system, they think of the *peripheral nervous system (PNS)*, a system of nerves that originates in the two large hemispheres of our brain, courses down the spinal cord, exiting through the spinal nerves, and runs peripherally throughout the body, innervating the musculoskeletal machinery of movement. It is this component of the nervous system that gives us the ability to throw a ball or experience the exquisite pain associated with jamming our funny bone when we clip our elbow on the corner of a table.

The ANS is a parallel and largely unappreciated component of our nervous system, which also courses throughout the body. The ANS, derived from the Greek *autonomos* meaning self-ruling, functions below our level of consciousness or intent and controls all homeostatic functions of the body. This homeostatic control is innate to all life and is, essentially, beyond control of the human will, other than perhaps in some very few Yogis and meditative adepts who are able to demonstrate ability to slow down respiration and pulse rates in a hibernation mode for extended periods of time.

The ANS's neurological homeostatic control defines the body's ability to maintain its internal equilibrium by altering physiological processes, essentially managing all the necessary internal environmental changes for execution of cellular life function. These physiological controls, which last as long as life is present, influence all organ functions including heart and lung performance, metabolic and digestive function and all endocrine organ systems.

The ANS is responsible for preserving all basic primordial functions as exemplified by maintenance of blood pressure at a steady state and control of thermoregulation by keeping body temperature stable in the face of wide swings of temperature in the surrounding environment.

How Stress Degrades Our Health; Recognizing the Symptoms of Stress

In a previous section, we learned how neuropathic pain can play havoc in the central nervous system, disrupting our pain recognition system, creating abnormal magnification and intensification alterations in this basic biological survival system. Chronic stress can equally disrupt the body's nervous system by interfering with the internal microenvironment of the ANS's regulatory control causing multiple-system maladaptive changes with widespread deleterious effects.

> An environment of chronic stress can derange almost any aspect of our autonomic nervous system

The human response to stress is an ancient physiological response inherited from our prehistoric ancestors. Since the initial studies in the last century by Hans Selye, the recognized father of research in stress studies, fewer areas in medical research have received more attention. Many reproducible studies have consistently demonstrated alterations in body function secondary to the effect of chronic stress.

When human beings are initially subjected to stress, the adrenal glands begin producing increased amounts of adrenaline, an influential neural hormone responsible for activating our body's defensive mechanisms. The elevated adrenaline levels cause, amongst other changes, an increase in heart rate and blood pressure, increased tension in our muscles and dilatation of our pupils—a cluster of body responses resulting in what is known as the physiological "fight or flight" response.

When stress is sustained over an extended period, the body responds by producing increasingly higher levels of cortisol, a stress hormone, which has significant biological effects on the maintenance of our internal homeostatic mechanisms. Persistence of elevated cortisol levels caused by chronic pain and stress may result in mood deregulation, cognitive impairment and even insulin resistance with alteration of blood sugar levels in otherwise healthy adults.

Most of these pathological manifestations come about because of disruption in the regulation of our ANS. Almost any aspect of this internal control can be deranged in an environment of chronic stress. As most people will have experienced stress at one time or another in their life, many of the widespread symptom complexes in the illustrated table that accompany stress will be recognizable.

As one can see from the long list of physical manifestations of stress, the ANS is involved in the biological control of widespread metabolic functions including liver metabolism, food digestion and kidney excretory function. Working in the background below our awareness, the ANS controls our skin and core temperature by sending messages to each blood vessel in the peripheral skin, producing contraction or dilation in the vessels in a complex system that preserves or allows escape of heat from the body. Blood pressure is similarly maintained by a delicate balance of neural transmission to microscopic muscles in each artery and vein, dilating or constricting each of them infinitesimally to produce an even blood pressure, ensuring a steady state of perfusion, sustaining life from moment to moment.

Symptoms of Stress

Physical Symptoms & Disorders	Emotional and Psychological Reactions	Changes in Behaviour
Heart palpitations	Frequent memory lapses	Increase in smoking
Muscle tension	Negative thinking	Increase in alcohol use
Headaches/migraines	Indecisiveness	Increase in use of prescribed
Loss of energy/fatigue	Lack of concentration	psychotropic drugs
Poor sleep patterns	Loss of libido	Increased use of street drugs
Grinding of teeth (bruxing)	Impatience	
Loss or increase in appetite	Impulsiveness	
High blood pressure	Hyperactivity	
Reduced resistance to	Aggressiveness	
infection	Anxiety	
Irritable Bowel Syndrome	Nervousness	
Ulcers	Worry	
Digestive disorders	Depression	
Heart attacks	Anger	
Angina	Irritability	
	Guilt	
	Moodiness	

The Inner World of Our Nervous System

The ANS performs neurological functions that have existed in living organisms since life began. Its nerve fibers originate deep in nuclei buried in the recesses of the primitive human brain, developing in the hypothalamus region where they are divided into two branches: the *sympathetic or adrenergic (adrenaline) branch* and the counteracting *parasympathetic (Vagal) branch*. Each of these two major branches of the ANS will course through the chest and abdominal cavities, as well as into the arms and legs, supplying nerve branches to every internal organ, glandular and vesicular structure in the body.

Much like the peripheral nervous system (PNS), controlling the motor movement of the body, has a division to gather sensory information to react to painful stimuli and proprioceptive information, the ANS also has a sensory information pathway, which serves as an internal intelligence system, returning continual feedback information to the brain where it is processed, sorted and acted upon, even during deep sleep.

> The work of the ANS is an interpretive dance of life, existing entirely below our level of awareness

The sensory information carried by the ANS allows the body to interpret information, both of the outer world as well as the microcosmic internal environment that bathes every living cell. This dynamic system of continual information streaming and simultaneous, reactive neural responses is an interpretive dance of life with constant, infinitesimal changes that mystically provide a steady, homeostatic state existing entirely below our level of awareness.

The two branches of the ANS (adrenergic and vagal) work in opposition to each other. For example, one branch will cause dilation of the blood vessels to lessen blood pressure while the opposite branch will cause constriction of the blood vessels to increase blood pressure. This opposing effect of the ANS will be applied to every organ and function to which it has input, balancing and regulating hormone production, digestion and all other regulatory functions of the body, creating a delicately balanced system reflecting the momentary needs of each individual organ, while at the same time overseeing the global, homeostatic status of the entire human body.

The ANS, therefore, behaves much like a "behind the scenes", executive director implementing on-going decisions, making sure that the business of the company carries on productively and in an uninterrupted manner, ensuring each department receives the necessary information on which to act, as well as the necessary resources to perform the tasks entrusted to it.

A healthy, regulated ANS maintains homeostasis, responding immediately and effectively with the necessary internal operational changes in response to the constantly changing stresses presented to our bodies. Each response must be gauged effectively and appropriately, reflecting the ability of the body to intelligently interpret the presenting stimuli.

A homeostatic change may be as simple as a need to adjust body temperature in response to increased physical exercise in a warm environment, or a considerably more complex response to a emergent, stressful challenge interpreted by the body as a "fight or flight" total body response when faced with imminent danger. In this latter situation, the end result may be decidedly complex depending on the urgency of the stimulus including, amongst other body responses, the necessary changes in respiratory and heart rates to match a possible need for immediate physical response. One can only be amazed at the widespread, homeostatic, reactive capabilities of the ANS, when it is pointed out that part of this whole body response includes dilation of the pupil of the eye to ensure the maximum amount of light enters the visual field, aiding in our visual scan for danger.

The ANS is responsible for regulatory function that extends to every endocrine-producing system throughout the body. Stress is capable of disrupting the ANS's influence on all of these organ systems. Included in this array of influence of the ANS are the adrenal glands, which produce cortisone, the major stress-regulating hormone; the thyroid gland, which produces thyroxine, a key regulating hormone, which acts as a watchdog over all others; and testosterone and estrogen, hormones that define our gender characteristics.

Biologically active hormones produced by the endocrine glandular structures within the body have distant, widespread effects on body functions. Some hormones act as neurotransmitters within the nervous system itself, facilitating effective and rapid transmission of neural impulses along the nerve pathways. Other hormone molecules function as circulating internal regulators, providing information and instructions to assist in regulatory control of distant organs. These hormones arrive on site by hitchhiking throughout our vascular system, piggybacked along with blood and other nutrients as they course through the vascular system, providing nourishment to each living cell.

> Chronic stress results in an eventual depletion of our body's resources and, ultimately, our health

Improving Posture Fends off Chronic Stress

Chronic stress results in an eventual depletion of our body's resources and in time decreases the ability of our defence systems in fending off threats to our health integrity. Chronic stress will make us vulnerable to illness and disease, as well as producing a host of emotional problems, leaving us with feelings of insecurity and inadequacy.

Our efforts to reduce chronic back pain will make substantial inroads in reducing stress patterns and their effect upon us. The effect of efforts at improving postural alignment and removing the burden of postural back pain sets the stage for an improved working environment for the autonomic nervous system. Reduction of pain and cessation of overactive stress hormone production allows homeostatic mechanisms to reset, permitting internal organ environments to re-establish normal, balanced function.

Alleviation of stress patterns and the restoration of normal metabolic, homeostatic mechanisms generates immediate, measurable results in restoration of a balanced and supportive biological environment. Measurable parameters showing improvement include return to normal regulation of blood sugars, lowering of cholesterol levels and return of normotensive blood pressures—all internal environmental changes which provide a milieu supporting a sustained and biologically balanced, healthy life.

Although there may arguably be other elements at play other than maintenance of ideal postural stance, studies in Western medicine have demonstrated systemic physiological changes that are clinically measurable in Taijiquan practitioners. Studies evaluating homeostatic controls of Taijiquan participants demonstrate evidence of higher levels of thyroid stimulating hormone, thyroid hormone and follicle stimulating hormone production in women when compared to control groups, evidential of biologically alert and responsive systems. Other researchers have demonstrated evidence suggesting that the postural control aided by Taijiquan exercises may extend healthy adult metabolic rates into advanced years, thereby retarding the biological aging process.

There is also evidence in the same subject group, that their body systems have the capability of increasing noradrenaline production, a neurotransmitter responsible for facilitating the electrical energy flow of nerve impulse transmission. These same subjects also show decreased salivary cortisol levels indicating a reduction in individual stress levels, a finding that may explain the observation of documented decreases in incidence of mood disorders and anxiety complaints in Taijiquan practitioners.

Our efforts to reduce chronic back pain will aid in reducing stress patterns

The presence of stress, even for short periods, is characteristically marked by a universally experienced loss of empowerment, with feelings of helplessness expressed in the struggle to deal with the constant stream of life's problems. This constant bombardment of new demands and our inability to meet expectations, both our own as well as those imposed on us, continue to feed the fire of helplessness, creating even greater levels of stress.

Understanding the dynamics of how stress begins and the effect it has on our body can help empower our own position by understanding what choices we can make to help us turn the tables and move in another direction—one that is focused on a successful outcome.

We have ample medical evidence to demonstrate that maintaining erect posture will result in reduction of pain, in itself a critical factor to reducing stress and producing positive effects in our basic homeostatic controls. We also have evidence that having made choices to work at maintenance of erect posture, we can bring about measurable biological change that will restore the homeostatic foundations of cellular health with far-reaching effects, both in our physical and emotional well-being.

Promise #6: Your Appearance Will Become More Athletic and Youthful with Increasing Levels of Fitness and Energy

12

P R O M I S E

An experienced clinician always places careful significance on the appearance of a patient entering into the examining room. Valuable clinical signs gleaned from the freedom of movement in the walk to the willingness to make eye contact, all help the physician piece together the holistic health picture that will assist in management of the patient's well-being. The carriage of a person and how they move is a window into the energy of that person and how comfortable they feel in their world right now. Not surprisingly, every time you meet someone you make the same assessment—as does everyone else!

Posture, Attractiveness and Natural Selection

It is innate to all of us to be cognizant of the health in people around us, recognizing those that are frail and unwell, as well as the healthy and vibrant. It is a matter of historical debate whether this natural sense is an intuitive characteristic borne from the instinct to choose superiorly healthy partners and avoid possible contamination with infectious diseases, or a quality that we develop out of altruistic behavior that makes us sympathetic to the plight of others, encouraging us as social beings to help our fellow man. The fact of the matter is, however, that it is an inborn talent in all of us.

Athleticism and good posture assume favorable prejudice in the hierarchy of attention

It has long been recognized in sociological studies that healthy appearances, attractiveness in facial features and the way we carry ourselves, are selectively rewarded in social circles as well as in the workplace. In classroom settings, teachers unwittingly keep eye contact far more with attractive students than those not considered attractive. Not surprisingly, promotion in the workplace can follow similar patterns, occasionally snubbing talent and competence.

It is almost embarrassing to find that even having been forewarned as to these prejudices, and as intelligent as we may consider ourselves, we all fall prey to the desire of wanting to be around attractive people. Most of us would be equally self-conscious if others were to be aware of the ministrations that we personally undertake, primping in our mirrors each morning in preparation of meeting the world.

This innate talent to pick out the superior specimens amongst us, especially those that embody athleticism and preservation of youth, creates interesting sociological observations in any age group, but particularly assumes a "bigger than life" social focus as we approach our middle-age years and compete for position in the corporate world.

Athleticism and good posture, like a good tan, have connotations and meanings that go beyond simple observation. A good tan, although indicative really only of exposure to perhaps too much sun, often carries additional connotations, implying without any proof, a general aura of well-being, rest and relaxation, an overall sense transmitted to the observer that this overbaked individual is enjoying particularly good health.

Athleticism and good posture, by the same token, assume favorable prejudice in the hierarchy of attention, a reflection of the value society places on youthfulness in our competitive social environment. Athleticism and youthfulness imply energy and power, qualities that we associate with the "fire in the belly" success orientation, and, therefore, seemingly good qualities to have associated with ourselves.

Although these theories, favorably reviewed in Victorian times, were debunked in the last century with the renaissance of reason in sociological study, they continue to influence judgment, often unfairly, with undue hardship to many unsuspecting individuals.

This same societal attitude to athleticism and vigor is also intimately associated with wardrobe fashions. Clothes were not designed on mannequins crumpled into poor postures. Mannequins are designed and constructed to reflect perfectly held postures; clothes are designed to fit mannequins, not slumped figures. It makes sense, therefore, that only those people maintaining upright, balanced postures will appreciably show off the current fashions of the day. No amount of money spent on exclusive designs will improve the look of the clothes on a figure that adopts a slouching attitude without any appreciable element of energy. The very best models have spent considerable time and expense in pursuit of "perfect posture" and the world responds in kind with adulation and a rush to purchase the carefully orchestrated display of fashions.

How Posture Changes can Enhance Fitness and Cardiovascular / Respiratory Efficiency

Fitness is not generally used as a medical term, for it does not describe the biological integrity of any one system, but incorporates a global, holistic evaluation of health and self-awareness, incorporating physical, emotional and mental characteristics. From a physical point of view, its implies features associated with endurance, strength, flexibility and coordination.

> Each incremental improvement in fitness begets more of the same

Diligent attention to good posture results in improved fitness as the body undergoes metamorphic change in response to the new ergonomic position. The adoption of proper posture with lessening of pain, the increase in core strength and stability, improvement in balance and coordination, enhancement of neurological function and homeostatic integrity, and a general increase in energy, all contribute to an overall improvement in individual health that we interpret under the heading of physical fitness.

Physical fitness will improve with any increase in physical activity. The change in lifestyle associated with improvement in pain levels naturally leads to a desire and interest to participate in more of the life activities around us. As a result, each incremental improvement in fitness begets more of the same.

Maintenance of correct shoulder and pelvic girdle posture also results in the maximal volumetric capacity for both the thoracic as well as abdominal cavities.

Efforts at maintaining upright postural stature supports chest wall architecture, preventing it from collapsing inward. A simple demonstration of this can be observed in the progressive dwindling of breath volume caused by bringing the shoulders forward, while leaning in and collapsing the chest cavity. Maintaining an upright posture creates maximal volumetric capacity in the thorax allowing the respiratory cycle to achieve greater tidal volumes, increasing lung inflation and improving respiratory exchange capacity.

The increased volume of the thoracic cavity also results in reduced pressure of the inflating lungs on the heart and great vessels, improving the heart's pump efficiency and blood circulation both in the lungs as well as in the peripheral circulation.

This same volumetric principle applies to the abdominal cavity, with the upright stature allowing freer movement of the diaphragm and decreasing downward pressure exerted on the liver, stomach and bowel. Adopting an upright stature with reduction of static pressure on the intestinal system, provides an environment for the intestines to perform an unrestricted, peristaltic movement. The reduced pressure aids digestion with minimal expenditure of effort and energy necessary to push the digesting food along the many yards of intestinal gut.

Both respiratory and cardiac benefits have been long documented in Taijiquan research reviews. It is somewhat surprising, however, to find improvement in these particular parameters in this study group, as there is no accompanying aerobic component in the Taijiquan form. Exercise studies, especially those examining exercise programs that involve aerobic components, exemplified by jogging, swimming or stair climbing, have always attributed the increased heart and respiratory rates as being the critical factors responsible for improvement in cardiovascular and respiratory performance. In the absence of any aerobic performance, the improvement in the Taijiquan group suggests that the improved postural stance in itself may be one of contributing factors resulting in improvements in these functional parameters.

How Improving Posture Increases Your Overall Energy

The question relating to improved energy is essentially an accounting issue. Energy means different things to different people. For one individual, energy may represent a measurable quantity defining the number of joules required to bring a beaker of water to boiling temperature; whereas, to another person, it represents an ethereal evaluation beyond physical absolutes, a concept central to a sense of well-being and transcending the absence of illness or disability.

> Surprisingly, it takes far more energy to support poor posture than it does perfect posture

For our purposes, let us define the *essential daily requirement of energy* as being that quantifiable bit of *"Oomph"* available to each of us, permitting accomplishment of our activities of daily living, and still having enough leftover to enjoy the other things we want to do in life.

We will, therefore, have a middle ground where the physical and emotional demands required of us are equal to the amount of energy that we are able to produce: a net even balance. From this middle ground, we can then have either a net increase or a net decrease value in available energy, dependent on the demands our body makes on the existing energy pool.

Many people will find it surprising to discover that it takes far more energy to support poor posture than it does perfect posture. Poor posture creates an imbalance in spinal alignment, necessitating overwork of at least some of the "shrouds and stays" representing core stabilization muscle systems, which have to do additional work in maintaining the upright axis of alignment against gravity. This represents work and expenditure of energy that would otherwise not be required if the spinal columnar segments were initially held correctly in upright posture.

Therefore, any correction of posture approaching the perfect posture model results in a net savings of energy expenditure, contributing to maintaining a net surplus in the total available energy pool.

Efforts at maintaining an erect and balanced posture, even for a small part of the day, result in sustained cardiorespiratory functional improvements, superior muscular strength and flexibility, and a heightened balance and poise.

Adoption of balanced posture results in significant physiological and psychosocial functional improvements with resilient resistance of the natural aging process. Maintenance of proper posture extenuates the characteristics of youthfulness and prevents decline in physical function, insuring an ability to maintain an active lifestyle that reaches into the upper percentiles of our relative peer groups.

Each successfully accomplished goal amplifies our personal confidence. The energy derived from these accomplishments continues to flame interest in further quests to exploit, while at the same time replenishing and maintaining, our youthful inner vigor.

The effect of postural balance enables reflections of athleticism and youthfulness and is a much-desired goal effectively reached with a small investment in effort. Commitments to enactment of our personal empowerment and a small outlay in energy directed towards the maintenance of an erect and balanced posture pays out in significant health benefits and dividends.

Reading Notes:

Promise #7:
You Will Awaken
Your Chong Mai

13

P R O M I S E

N o discussion on posture can be considered complete without reference to the contributions of traditional Chinese medicine (TCM) and Qi meridian theory. The correct attainment of posture is of such great importance in the maintenance of health in Chinese medicine, that the ancient teachers identified a single "extraordinary meridian" responsible for it.

How the Ancient Chinese Found the Qi of Perfect Posture

This meridian, called *Chong Mai*, endows the structure and foundation for the entire vertical axis of the body, starting at the feet and moving upward through our pelvic floor supporting the organs of the abdomen, and then extending upward through the spinal canal into the brain where it maintains a presence in the upper recesses of the intellect.

The complete practice of Chinese medicine focuses around the existence of Qi, the life energy that exists in all of us and is responsible for maintenance of life. Much like Eskimos define many different types of snow with detailed descriptions of its various characteristics, the Chinese differentiate many different types of Qi, all of which are responsible for maintenance of the various qualities of life.

One of the earliest Qi's endowed to us is the foundational energy of *Yuan Qi*, described as an inherited primal energy of life, a vitality transferred from one generation to the next, representing our inherited genetic endowment and very much active in the meridian of Chong Mai.

Another type of Qi known as *Wei Qi*, also described as Guardian Qi, manifests in the body periphery of the skin and muscles. This

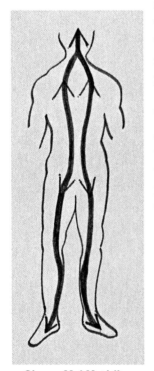

Qi serves as a defensive Qi and is responsible for warding off the many invasive forces, such as infectious agents, that bombard us daily and, if not defended against, would otherwise cause harm by disrupting the internal harmony of our body functions.

These various forms of Qi responsible for defence and maintenance of life, flow continuously through the meridians that completely envelop us. In addition to these peripheral highways of Qi, there are central reserve pools, which exist to provide additional Qi that can be quickly mobilized during moments of crisis, providing the necessary defence and support required.

Chong Mai Meridian

These reserve pools of Qi, referred to as "extraordinary vessels or meridians", describe an energetic organization that is present from the very moment of conception. They represent an organizational matrix of energy active from the earliest multicellular stages of fetal development, remaining critical throughout life, coordinating the necessary biological activities of the body and assisting in homeostatic equilibration and maintenance of a balanced life.

The term "extraordinary" is a somewhat inadequate attempt at English translation, an effort to convey the special importance of the role that these reserve pools play in supporting the subservient peripheral meridians, maintaining the smooth flow of energetic Qi and prevention of lapses in defence.

Of this group of extraordinary meridians, Chong Mai is considered paramount, directed with the responsibility for maintenance of the body's internal vertical axis. Along with these other extraordinary meridians, Chong Mai is responsible for linking the internal and external structural meridians contributing to the natural harmony and balance of the body's energetic system. The organization and administration of these energy systems result in a complete body unification of the dynamically active axial, longitudinal and equatorial energy matrixes.

In the diagrammatic representation of this meridian, Chong Mai is illustrated as beginning its roots at the feet, moving upward through the center of the axialskeletal spine and terminating in the internal recesses of the brain, where the Qi it brings energizes and nourishes the brain as well as the *Shen*, a word probably best described in English as the life energy representing the Inner Soul.

The Matrix of Our Inner Energy and the Energy that Surrounds Us

Chong Mai, in TCM, conceptually represents a global energy or vitality, an inner energy that is continuous with the external energy that surrounds us, rather than any particularly specific biological system as defined by Western medicine.

While this conceptualization of Chong Mai recognizes the prerequisite of a healthy and balanced biological system for its manifestation, it additionally addresses the existential and metaphysical component that encompasses every living organism, identifying the need for that organism to interact with the energy of the environment surrounding it to maintain its existence.

Chinese medicine believes that we as individuals, as do all living creatures, form a part of this greater picture and the global energy matrix. Our own inner energy participates in this ballet, dynamically moving in and out of the energy matrix surrounding it—

sometimes giving, sometimes receiving, but never completely separate or distinct.

Western cultures also recognize a similar relational energy connected to life, transcending the physical realm. For example, as expressed in the French language, *joie de vivre* is descriptive language that portrays the joy that accompanies a well-celebrated life, free and animated, distinct from the physical or emotional encumbrances that are part and parcel of each individual life.

Kuo Lien Ying ... Holding the Ball
Photographer and Family Contacts Unknown

Chinese medical texts frequently use eloquent, metaphorical language in the classical writings, giving the reader a distinct feeling for each specific meridian. In ancient literature, Chong Mai is referred to as "the Mother of the internal organs" and "the sea of the principal meridians", connotations suggesting a primordial force. The energy description of Chong Mai is considered Yin and maternal, nourishing all the internal organs responsible for maintaining life, and the complicated internal homeostasis that governs the body's overall balance of energy flow.

In contemporary Western medical terms, we would say that Chong Mai is responsible for the endocrine hormonal axis, providing energy that maintains sexual energy and reproductive function, excretory function of kidney and bladder, the various functions of metabolism and digestion, and the maintenance of vigor and power provided by cardiorespiratory function. The Chong Mai's meridian system is responsible for linking all these executive life functions with the brain, where the meridian branches penetrate deep

134

into the recesses of the brain linking the endocrine-feedback regulatory centers.

In addition to its somatic responsibilities and functions, Chong Mai has a role in its contribution to the metaphysic and holistic model of health, with responsibilities supporting the psycho-emotional components of overall health.

Nourishing the Chong Mai Energy System

If we expect to draw upon the energy of Chong Mai or any other meridian, it is equally realistic that we must nourish the meridian to maintain its vitality so that this energy is available to us when we require it.

In addition to the use of acupuncture, this can be accomplished through specific Qigong physical exercises designed to massage the structural axial core muscles of the spine, thereby promoting the flow of energy in the Chong Mai meridian. In this practice, specific techniques of movement and breathing are employed to facilitate the movement of Qi throughout the various branches of its complex meridian pattern. Particular attention is paid to maintaining perfect posture during the practice of Qigong, for it is a basic tenet of Chinese medicine that, without attention to posture, the flow of energy within the meridian is sluggish and obstructed.

> Even the most hardened scientists recognize that human health is more than just the absence of disease

Nourishing the Chong Mai is essential, not only in the principles of traditional Chinese medicine, but in Taoist spiritual training as well, where the same principles of Qigong are used in the practice of mindful cultivation, along the journey of enlightenment.

135

The nourishment of Chong Mai in Taoist practices is accomplished by regulation of breathing combined with profound meditative states, energizing the brain cells to a higher level of focus and concentration, with the ultimate goal of nourishing the Shen (Inner Soul) and opening the intuitive third eye.

There is recognition even amongst the most hardened scientists that human health represents more than just the absence of disease. It is an acknowledgment that human health represents a sense of well-being: physically and emotionally, as well as metaphysically. It is an appreciation that each individual's life energy cannot exist independent of the energy that surrounds that life.

Each life, and the energy that is associated with it, must interact with the environment encircling it, blurring the distinction of individuality. Chinese medicine, respectful of this *mist of quantum continuum*, has recognized this relationship between "local and global" from the time of early writings.

In TCM, the practice of perfect posture and the nourishment of the Chong Mai meridian are inseparable

Although the concept of Chong Mai may be ethereal, the application of maintaining its vitality is far more straightforward in the practice of Chinese medicine. It is the observance of the postural standards as practiced in Qigong and Taijiquan that promote the health and vigor of Chong Mai.

In Chinese medicine, the practice of perfect posture and the nourishment of the Chong Mai meridian are inseparable and have to do with *connectedness*—both to what is happening within us, as well as to what is happening in the environment around us. It is a sensory awareness maintained consciously and subconsciously, intellectually and intuitively, working simultaneously on both a biological and ethereal plane.

The postural standards of erectness allow freedom of movement and a sensory alertness that allows immediate, anticipatory action. For those privileged adepts, there is the promise of enlightenment after decades of diligent practice and the pledge of sensory wholeness with the universal energy that surrounds us.

For the rest of us, Chong Mai represents a lifetime journey celebrated by small but measurable milestones in the manifestation of our personal empowerment towards attainment of perfect posture and all its promises.

Reading Notes:

PART III

THE 7 SECRETS OF PERFECT POSTURE

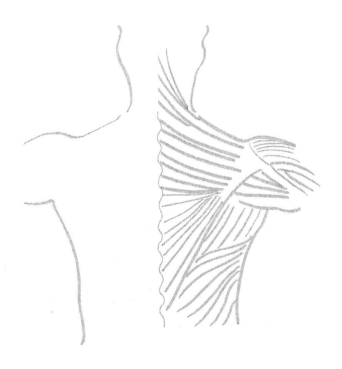

The Mental Imagery of Posture

The lack of anatomical illustrations and visual guides in teaching postural alignment is a deliberate training strategy rather than an oversight. The reason is that ideal postural alignment is specific to each individual, starting from wherever you are now and moving in a direction developed in the mind's eye through intent and focus.

The Individual Fingerprint of Perfect Posture

For each of us, postural alignment will have the individuality of a fingerprint or snowflake, determined by our bone structure, our muscles and our ligaments in terms of strength and malleability, as well as the energy that we have at any given time. It is, therefore, impossible to instruct an individual to copy the appearance of a model in the pursuit of ideal posture with any hope of success.

Illustrations may actually interfere with the mental imagery necessary to find ideal posture because they present suppositions, which may otherwise unhelpfully influence the conscious workings necessary to allow our body to find the proprioceptive benchmark that represents our moment of postural balance. For posture is all about balance, that sense of *"middleness"* that, given the opportunity, our proprioceptive neurophysiology will seek out and find.

There is far more success in working towards ideal postural alignment by instilling imagery, allowing the structural concepts to be built in our visual cortex and then, finally, through focused intention integrated into our postural foundation. Whereas in many teaching situations *a picture is worth a thousand words,* when it comes to teaching kinesthetic imagery, language is probably a more effective paint, with verbal instruction to the individual taking the place of pictures in transmitting the foundational concepts of posture.

> Language is a more effective paint in teaching kinesthetic imagery and the concepts of posture

Using kinesthetic imagery to reinforce and integrate models of postural alignment is not a new teaching tool and has been used extensively in dance, athletic pursuits, yoga and martial arts since antiquity. Our bodies, given the opportunity, find it much easier to react to imagery—especially when grasping the concepts of postural alignment.

How the Mind Creates Perfect Posture

The ability of the mind to direct the body using imagery skills needs to be developed, however, similarly to training in any other skill set that we are attempting to assimilate. Unlike strength training, which will predictably produce consistent improvement with classical straightforward programming, this may not necessarily be so with mental imaging.

The learning process of imagination may take more or less time than we think, because this mental integrative process is different for each individual. It is much easier to describe how a person walks than how they think, because there is a lack of consistency between how different individuals tackle mental problems. Whereas one individual may pick up imagery skills faster than another, in the end, we will all generally achieve the same skill level.

It is, therefore, necessary to allow your mind to remain more open when tackling some of these verbal instructions. In some cases, letting your mind mull over the visual offering, much like a dog gnawing on a bone in front of a warm fireplace, produces the best results.

It is always best with imagery to be playful and exploratory, a reason why children are generally better at it than adults. At first, our minds will mostly tend to be overly judgmental, worrying whether or not we are doing it correctly or if we are getting enough out of the exercise to justify persisting. We can even feel foolish because simple instructions may initially draw a blank, resulting in minimal effects. The best universal advice is to suspend judgment and give it a chance. Our mind hardly ever responds like a boot camp trainee taking orders from a drill instructor.

It is almost always easier, in the beginning, if imagery is practiced with our eyes closed; but, with time, we will become equally proficient performing the imagery exercises with our eyes open, effortlessly taking instructions from our conscious mind. It comes as a welcome surprise to find how quickly our mind catches on to what we are asking it to do.

Intention and motivation, as well as trusting the images, creates crystal clear impressions in our mind, making kinaesthetically directed exercise a rewarding experience and giving us the precise proprioceptive clues for which we are searching. Not surprisingly, our body will know when we get there—*it just feels right!*

Reading Notes:

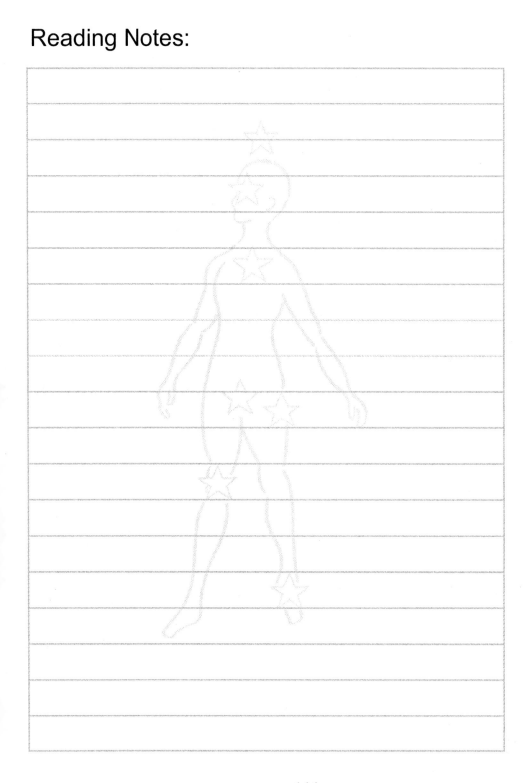

The 1st Secret: Trust Your Feet and Let Them Relax

15

T he evolutionary breakthrough in man's journey through time must certainly be related to the ability to achieve an upright bipedal stance, a moment defining a critical anthropomorphic milestone and one of the premier engineering marvels of nature.

The human body's ability to maintain upright balance, not only at rest but continuously during movement, with the body able to moderate its center of balance independently over each foot, constantly readjusting the integral structures within the foot and ankle to facilitate the changing axial line of gravity, reflects a neurological computing ability that modern artificial intelligence can only dream about.

A "Simple" Tripod Made Up of 26 Bones & 25 Joints

This ability to adapt to the changing center of gravitational balance begins in the complex structural foundation of the foot and ankle. Together, the foot and ankle encompass 26 bones forming 25 individual component joints, making up a shifting, dynamic set of arches over a stable pod. This complicated bioengineering model permits minute, multiple tension adjustments to support not only stable and stationary weight, but to also provide the ability to adapt to changing vector forces and pressure loads caused by transitional movement.

The foot is essentially a tripod with pressure points at the first and fifth toes and the heel

With the practice of wearing shoes from a very early age, most of us have been robbed, over time, of the ability to appreciate the sensitive capabilities of our feet to read the terrain upon which we are walking. The structural integrity of shoes also negates the necessity for the foot and ankle to perform many of the complex movements otherwise necessary, while, for example, running barefoot along uneven trails, with the natural undulations of the ground underfoot.

In order to appreciate "The 1st Step to Perfect Posture" involving the complex multiple movements within the foot and ankle unit, and their contribution to our postural foundation, it is probably best to practice walking barefoot, appreciating the subtle joint movements of the foot and ankle both on flat as well as on uneven surfaces.

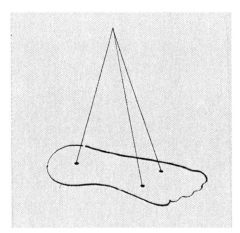

The first thing to appreciate is that the foot is essentially a tripod with the weight-bearing pressure points situated at the base of the first and fifth toes and, at the back, on the base of the heel. The second thing that we can appreciate is that the foot is divided into three contiguous and interacting sections, each of which has a specific task to perform in the maintenance of overall stability of the postural root.

146

The Three Separate, Interacting Parts of the Foot:

The Hind-Foot

The hind-foot is comprised of the two bones forming the heel, the talus and the calcaneus. The hind-foot forms the base of this tripod and when firmly planted on the ground provides the greatest single surface contact of the foot with the **ground**, thereby being the major contributor to stability of stance.

The Mid-Foot

The mid-foot is formed by the tarsal bones, a diverse group of irregularly shaped bones, enclosed together within a ligamentus sack. This enclosed group of bones behaves much like a bag of irregularly shaped pebbles, which, when dropped, has the ability to rearrange and mould itself to an irregularly shaped surface on which it has fallen, conforming to the axial plane without sliding off in one direction or another. It is this function of the mid-foot, which gives the lower leg the capability of staying centrally balanced over the planted foot. The mid-foot section of bones also provides the arch system to the foot, giving the foot and ankle the capability of spring, thrust and shock absorbance.

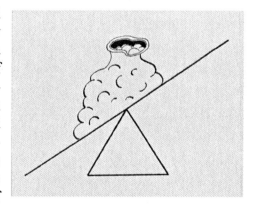

The Fore-Foot

The fore-foot is comprised of the toes (phalanges) and the long bones (metatarsals) leading up to them—14 bones in all. Each of the long bones in the fore-foot has the ability to move independently of each other. Like individual logs composing a river raft, each metatarsal bone can roll and twist up and down along its axis,

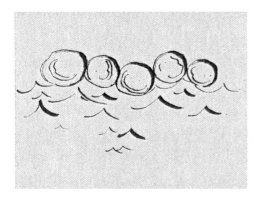

adapting to the changes of uneven terrain underfoot, much like a raft of loosely tied logs negotiating a stretch of rapids

The fore-foot also has the ability to do this independently from the mid-foot, adjusting to changes in terrain, while the mid-foot and hind-foot work together, forming a solid mortise for the weight of the body supported above.

Another notable characteristic of the foot is that its outside edge provides the primary support surface with the underlying terrain, while its inside edge provides the supporting archways and spring

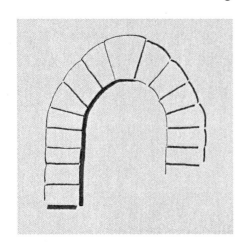

capabilities. Architecturally, the arch of the foot has the appearance of a vaulted cupola in a cathedral window inserted into a thick stone wall. Different bands of ligamentous tissue run multi-directionally through the roof, providing the buttressing strength necessary to support the overlying weight.

The floor of the arch of the foot is supported by a strong fascial band, which runs longitudinally along the length of the bottom of the foot and provides spring to the foot, much like the bow string on an inverted, medieval archer's bow.

How the Versatile Ankle Mortise Gives Us the First and Most Important Foundation of Balance

Sitting directly above the foot is the ankle mortise comprised of the pillar bones (tibia and fibula), which balance themselves over the mid-foot collection of enclosed tarsal bones. This pillar is positioned slightly back from the center of the foot and, with the assistance of the muscles controlling the ankle, is able to dynamically shift over the center of gravity running up through the foot.

The delicate changes in balance in the ankle, necessary for upright bipedal stance, are much the same as in the childhood trick of balancing a broomstick on an open palm, moving the hand in whichever direction is necessary to keep the broomstick upright in the air.

> One half of all Qi energy meridians take root in the foot, drawing energy form the earth

In addition to the obvious flexion movements of the ankle, allowing the toe to point downward as well as upward, it also has the capability to invert inwardly and outwardly, allowing the foot to pronate and supinate, both positions which can be seen when standing behind someone and watching them make their way down the length of a pitched roof.

Whereas, at first, we might visualize the foot as only a simple pad upon which to place our body weight, we can now see how it becomes a complex structural pod capable of an almost infinite combination of structural movements and balance adjustments, neurologically orchestrated as we negotiate the varied surfaces upon which we walk.

Why in Chinese Medicine All the "Emergency 911" Acupuncture Points are in the Foot

The role of the foot and its contribution to the status to which man rises in the hierarchy of the animal kingdom was not lost on the ancient Chinese. The medical "Ancients" of Chinese history, in recognition of the foot's contribution to the evolutionary ascendance of mankind, dictated that one half of all primary Qi energy meridians would take root in the foot, drawing on energy from the earth upon which we walk.

The significance of this assignment becomes meaningful when one realizes that the other half of all the primary Qi energy meridians begin in the hand, reflecting another critical evolutionary landmark of mankind. The capability of grasping and manipulating tools with our opposable thumb, allowing the hand to grasp objects between the thumb and each of the fingers with infinitesimal sensitivity, provided man with a giant step in control of his environment.

> "Jing Well" acupuncture points are considered to be among the most powerful of all

In addition to the dozens of acupuncture points situated on the foot, utilized in the treatment of global, systemic medical problems, the foot is also home to the "Jing Well" points situated at the end of the toes. These seminal acupuncture points are considered to be among the most powerful of all therapeutic intervention acupoints, and are extremely important in the treatment of medical emergencies including hemorrhage, strokes, shock and loss of consciousness.

Many specific foot-massage techniques were developed in traditional Chinese medical treatments to impart healing energy to the major organ systems. Modern Western Complementary Medical Therapies, as exemplified by reflexology, have also evolved to encompass similar therapeutic strategies.

All this attention given to the *lowly foot* by preceding civilizations, should make us wonder if perhaps we take the foot too much for granted, underestimating its contribution to our postural integrity.

The Paradox of Perfect Posture and Relaxing Your Feet —the More You Relax, the Easier It Is

So, how can we apply all this information to help us establish the very best postural foundation with our feet? The answer, surprisingly, will not come from increasing our physical effort because, ironically, our foundational root can only be improved by relaxation of the foot. A conscious effort to relax the intrinsic muscles of the foot permits the toes to reach forward and spread out, giving the plantar aspect of the foot the maximal contact with the underlying terrain.

Have you ever noticed that when you are very tense, you tend to unconsciously curl your toes in a tense, clenching fashion, much like you might clench your fists under similar circumstances? Can you imagine trying to run or even walk with such tension in your feet? It is easy to see then that relaxation of the feet is critical for relaxation of the body.

Relaxation of our feet remains such a strong signal to the rest of the body that in some sports, like golf, you will see professionals prepare for a putt by deliberately lifting their fore-foot to spread and stretch the toes to relax the feet. They will also bounce on their heels, allowing the relaxation sensation to ripple up their bodies to the shoulders and neck, freeing up the muscular tension so the arc of the putting stroke will be true and free of stress in the controlling shoulder girdle muscles.

Applying "The 1st Secret of Perfect Posture" involves appreciating the complicated role of our feet and ankles in adapting to the terrain on which we are standing and walking, and trusting them to do the job for which they were designed.

Ironically, our foundational root can only be improved by *relaxation* of the foot

We can do this in only one way: by making a conscious effort to relax the small muscles controlling movement in the foot and ankle, trusting our feet to find the foundational support intrinsic to a stable postural stance.

Application Exercises

Bounce on your heels until you can feel the relaxation ripple like a wave up through the body to your shoulder girdle and neck.

Alternately curl and stretch your toes while at the same time keeping your weight back on your heels and lifting your fore-foot off the floor.

Walk slowly, barefoot, over uneven surfaces or, better yet, on moving surfaces like a floating dock, paying attention to the adjustments your ankles and feet must make to the changing environment.

Walk barefoot as much as possible, or in stocking feet or moccasins, to gain an appreciation of the intrinsic movements of the small foot muscles—changes we don't appreciate when wearing shoes.

Develop an awareness of your central axis of gravity situated directly over your ankles and spreading inferiorly like fingers stretching into the dynamic arches of the mid-foot. We can do this by standing like a heron or a Masai warrior on one leg, appreciating the multiple intrinsic movements occurring in the foot and ankle in the process of maintaining balance.

Perform small jumps up and down to experience the spring in the arches of your feet, making a conscious effort to relax the muscles in the arch of the foot as you feel the give in your feet supporting the weight of your landing body.

The 2nd Secret: Feel the Springboard in Your Knees

The knees might be one of the great, unsung heroes in the discussion of human joint anatomy. While it is common to have people talk about their knees if they experience a problem with them, it is rare and highly unlikely that someone will spontaneously proclaim how terrific their knees feel! In fact, this may be reflective of our appreciation of health in general, with the "bits and pieces" of us that work unerringly well receiving little notice until the system fails, at which time it consumes our undivided attention.

The Knee Is the Largest and Most Powerful Joint in the Body

The knee is not only the largest joint in the human body but likely the joint most associated with powerful acceleration, power generated by the most robust muscles in the human body: those that surround and encompass the thigh.

The ability of the knee to lever this powerful propulsion is beautifully illustrated in the travelogue scenes of the African Serengeti, with springbok antelope springing almost vertically and then bouncing off in great, effortless leaps and bounds, disappearing into the distant horizon.

As long as our knees do not give us any trouble, most of us give little thought to the complicated function of this hinge arrangement. More than likely, the only attention afforded this structure up to now was our passing interest in the familiar sight of the bottom end of a chicken drumstick.

"I think if I were God, I might have designed the knee joint a little differently."

This familiar knucklebone-end of the drumstick is the top half of the knee, with the bottom articulating surface of the knee represented by the upper surface of the tibial plateau, which is exactly how it looks: a flat-topped mountain Mesa, such as seen in a desert cartoon drawing.

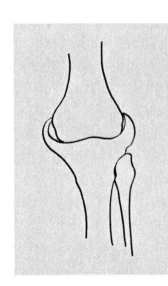

What keeps the knuckles from sliding to one side or another are the meniscal plates; bumper guards that form a circumferential guard rail running along the outside of the supporting tibial plateau. In addition to the medial and lateral meniscii guard rails contributing to the lateral stability of the knee, there are two cruciate ligaments arising within the knee joint itself and connecting the two bones of the knee, providing stability in the "fore and aft" direction.

Why the Most Powerful Joint Is Also the Most Vulnerable Joint in the Athlete

On first glance, the knee gives the appearance of a ball sitting upon a table—-a very tenuous structure indeed to support the entire body weight. In fact, as one first-year bioengineering student said as he looked at a model of the knee joint, "I think if I were God, I might have designed this joint a little differently."

Unlike the hip or shoulder, which have large masses of muscle supporting and holding the joint tightly in place, the knee is sitting right out there with little other than the streamlined tendons that surround it and the thin skin overlying it accounting for its integral support against the stresses of bending, thrusting and twisting, all movements associated with normal knee joint function.

It is the streamlined design and functionality of this joint, however, that also gives the knee its intimate association with athleticism. In spite of its great power and role in athletic balance, it is not surprising, because of its design, to find that the knee is also one of the most commonly injured joints in sports, especially when these sports involve competitive body contact.

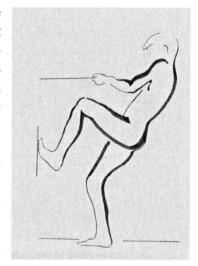

The knee's ability to withstand force vectors from the side comes up against rigid bioengineering limits. The resultant sports-related injuries, as are often seen in competitive athletes, lead to lengthy convalescence periods with the possibility of permanent, crippling injuries and disabilities that can plague them into their advanced years.

Why the Knee Is the Second Most Important Contributor to Balance

In addition to its great power, the knee also plays a major contributory role to balance, an attribute equally unappreciated.

Much like the role of the ankle as it strives to get underneath the weight of the overlying tibial bone, the knee—even more importantly—must get underneath the weight of the upper body in order to maintain a center of balance. In fact, failure of the knees to get under the body's weight inevitably results in a fall unless the individual has the necessary agility and strength to recover the loss of gravitational balance by sliding the knees back under the body's weight.

In order to appreciate the role of the knee in providing foundational balance, it is necessary to look beyond the obvious hinge movement the knee provides. The knee is capable of a slight twisting rotation, which is more obvious when the knees are slightly bent than when fully extended in a locked position.

With this simple tip, you can exercise your knees with no risk

It is this ability to make minute, radial adjustments to react to incoming vector forces, that gives the knee its capability of almost infinite movement combinations, allowing it to maintain a center of balance under the overlying body. In this regard, the balanced knee provides a foundation for the thighbone in much the same balanced fashion as illustrated earlier by the "upright broomstick balancing act".

In actual fact, unless we keep this slight bend in our knees, we completely lose this ability to make these minute adjustments in balance, instead taking on the appearance of the stiff gaited stance of the circus clown walking on stilts. This is often the gait we see in elderly people who are at risk of falling, situations that develop from chronic wasting conditions of muscles in the upper thigh, with the resultant difficulty in controlling movement at the knees and ability to support the foundational balance required in upright bipedal stance.

We can now see what a powerful yet responsive biomechanical engineering marvel the knee is, providing us with "The 2nd Secret of Perfect Posture": a critical, structural, anatomical device that enables us to fine tune our balance in the attainment of foundational support.

Protecting the Knee Against Injury

You will always hear the warning caveats about knee exercises: unless done correctly, one might expect aggravation of pre-existing knee injuries or even creation of new ones. This is advice that is certainly prudent to heed.

In all of these exercises it is very important, while bending the knee, that the front of the knee never extends forward beyond the second toe. (Hint: visualize your knee from the side.) By keeping your hands on your knee caps during all of these knee-bending exercises, and by keeping your eyes on the back of your hands, you can rest assured that you are well within the safety zone and risk no injury to your knees—if you can always see your toes extending past your view of your hands.

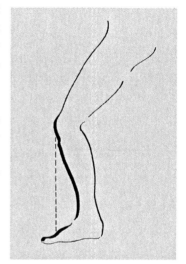

Application Exercises

Stand with your feet shoulder width apart and slowly make small jumps into the air—no more than one to two inches off the floor. Take plenty of time after each jump to let the neurological sensations of propelling the jump, and cushioning the subsequent landing, catch-up to your conscious mind, allowing it to appreciate the driving power as well as the gentle shock absorption provided by the knees on each jump.

Practice walking with the knees bent in a half sitting crouch to appreciate the immense strength existing in our thigh muscles—strength that provides us with both the ability of propulsion as well as shock absorption.

When you think no one is looking, skip a few steps like a carefree child or walk slowly, bouncing off your heels and up onto your toes with each step. Feel the strength of the great thigh muscles powering the springboard of the knee joint.

Stand upright in a locked knee position and slowly twist from side to side, feeling the hard endpoints preventing rotation. Now, very slowly, progressively bend the knees and again begin the twisting movement, recognizing the increasing scope of twisting movement permitted by bending the knees.

Put your hands on your kneecaps and, with your knees slightly bent, slowly move your knees in a circle parallel to the floor, spiralling out from very small circles to increasingly greater circles, and then working back again in a counterclockwise direction from big circles to increasingly smaller circles. Appreciate the ability of the knees to move in any direction and find almost any position necessary to move them under a dynamically changing gravitational axial line, as the upper body athletically stays centered above them.

The 3rd Secret: Keep Your Pelvis Tipped up

The pelvis, or pelvic girdle as it is often referred to, is a word taken from the Latin derivative meaning *basin*. Architecturally, the pelvic girdle resembles an open basin, with a bony brim and sides and a soft pelvic diaphragmatic floor supporting the lower abdominal contents.

Protecting the pelvic and lower abdominal organs, the two sides of the bony pelvis are joined together at the front with a fibrous connection called the *symphysis pubis*, and at the back where the pelvis forms the sacroiliac joints, with the wedge-shaped sacrum forming the base of the spine.

The Center of Movement Is in the Pelvis

The pelvic girdle also serves as the structural foundation for the root of the spinal column. The back of the pelvic girdle forms a cleft or saddle into which the sacrum articulates, forming the sacroiliac joints. Fitting like a wedge, the sacrum forms the foundational root from which the spinal column arises. The ability for the pelvic girdle to maintain a level platform and provide this stable foundation for the start of the spinal column remains critical, for as any carpenter will attest, "You cannot build a straight house on a crooked foundation."

From the standpoint of movement dynamics, the pelvic basin represents the central axis of gravity for the entire body.

All directional movement must start with a gravitational shift of the center of the pelvic girdle.

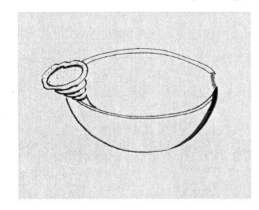

This universal principle is observed in martial arts as well as in all competitive sporting activities in which players attempt to disguise their movement intentions. Consider a forward trying to get past a defensive player: coaches advise to always watch the hips. In spite of what devious feints the advancing player may make, the hips and, therefore, the pelvic girdle movement will give away the true intention every time.

As an intermediary structure between the upper and lower body, the pelvic girdle also serves as a relay station for the forces traveling up through the legs as well as downward through the torso and into the legs. In addition to its role in movement initiation and coordination, the pelvic girdle, therefore, serves as a critical structure in modulating physical stresses on the body's axial skeletal structure.

The pelvic sacral plexus is considered by many leading physiologists to be a "second brain"

Why the Pelvis Is the Center of Life in Eastern Teachings

Because of its importance as a center of postural integrity, the pelvic girdle has been attributed important innate, spiritual values and sacredness in different Eastern philosophies in which the pelvic girdle is believed to house critical energy centers contributing to the mystical "center of life".

From a physiological point of view, even in Western medicine, there is a consideration that the pelvic basin may hold special significance in housing the pelvic sacral plexus, a collection of nerve ganglions that is considered by many leading physiologists to be a "second brain", attributed with autonomous powers in controlling the physiology of gut function. This special intelligence has even made it into the lexicon of the English language where we refer to a "gut feeling" in reference to a deep feeling we have relating to the certainty or genuineness of a given situation.

Dan Tian is considered the root and origin of our physical and spiritual lives

In Indian Tantric teachings, the pelvic girdle is home to two of the seven Chakras, known by their Sanskrit names as Muladhara and Svadhisthana. The first Chakra, Muladhara, is associated with stillness, security and stability, and is a critical foundational support for survival and grounding. The second Chakra, Svadhisthana, is intimately associated with the organs enclosed within the pelvic girdle serving the functions of procreation and sexuality. This is also the center of being that is associated with emotion and the gut feeling previously referred to as the "second brain".

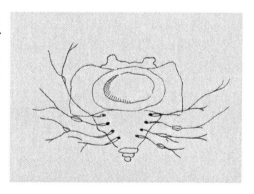

In Traditional Chinese medicine, the pelvic girdle is home to the Dan Tian, an important reservoir of Qi. Respected and revered for over 2,000 years by Buddhists, Taoists and martial artists alike, the Dan Tian is considered the root and origin of our physical and spiritual lives, and the Yang pole of the two opposite polarities that constitute the body's central energy system. Surprisingly enough, although substantially identified by a completely separate culture, the Dan Tian is responsible for the integrity of the same foundational life-support systems as acknowledged in Indian Tantric teachings.

How the Pelvis Moves and Why
It Is Important to Postural Stability

Like the ankle and knees, the pelvic girdle must also position itself under the weight of the torso in order to provide the foundation support of postural integrity. Much as the ankles and knees have to demonstrate the ability to position themselves under their overlying weight, the pelvic girdle is the last in this string of pearls that must achieve the same dynamics of movement assisted by the hips to prevent the body from falling or tipping while erect.

The range of motion of the pelvic girdle can be visualized as one might expect from a basin resting on the table surface. Recognizing that the basin has a rounded base, it may tip in any given direction. In fact, during movement of the pelvic girdle, observation of these subtle movements can be seen with careful monitoring.

For best postural stability, however, the basin should be kept level and if visualized filled with water, the pelvic girdle should continuously strive to keep the basin level without tipping any of its fluid contents during rest or with movement. The most likely direction of tipping the pelvis and spilling of its contents is forward, for both the back as well as the sides of the pelvic girdle are fixed firmly in place with their supporting bony ramparts. Therefore, our attention must only be necessarily kept on keeping the front brim of the pelvis supported up.

By keeping the pelvis level, we ensure that the weight of the overlying torso is balanced over the center of the pelvic girdle, providing the necessary postural stability and foundational support.

So, what muscles provide the integral support that keeps the pelvic girdle level and the pelvic brim tipped up? With most of us, the first muscle group that will come to mind are the abdominal muscles. These very strong muscles take their insertion from the bottom of the ribs and course downwards in different directional, powerful straps, both obliquely as well as vertically, from where they eventually attach to the front brim of the pelvis. By contracting our abdominal muscles and moving our belly button backwards (towards the front of our spine), we can create the effect of lifting the brim of the pelvis—but not without a cost.

The more we contract our abdominal muscles, the more difficult it is to effectively breathe because we limit the downward excursion of the diaphragm separating the chest from the abdominal contents, effectively embarrassing our respiratory efforts.

> **The psoas muscle serves as an important surgical sentinel sign for disease**

So, although the abdominal muscles provide a significant support keeping the front brim of the pelvis up, it is another major muscle, the psoas, that provides the major contribution to the effort of pelvic stabilization.

How One Muscle (Psoas Muscle) Does Most of the Work and Works like a Pair of Internal Suspenders

The psoas muscle, composed of the large psoas major and a smaller psoas minor, takes its insertion from the front of each of the lumbar vertebral backbones starting where the rib cage ends, running down through the back of the pelvis, inserting into the front brim of the pelvis and exiting through the groin to attach to the inner aspect of the upper thigh.

It has an intimate relationship, lying alongside all the major, important structures of the abdomen and pelvis, including the kidneys and the ureters draining them, the large gut, the great blood vessels and the spinal nerves, and the autonomic nerve ganglion complexes. For this reason, in acute surgical diagnosis, the psoas muscle serves as a very important medical sentinel sign for diseases of organs that lay alongside it, producing exquisite irritation and discomfort during examination, helping the surgeon identify the source of pathology.

The microscopic architecture of the psoas muscle is marked differently in bipedal humans than it is in four-footed creatures. The

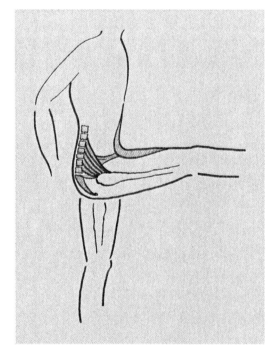

evolution of man to bipedal stance resulted in significant architectural changes in the psoas muscle fiber types. Whereas, in quadruped animals, the psoas muscle shows greater populations of Type 1 fibers (identified by smaller size, longer endurance, but less force capacity), upon assimilation of bipedal stance, the psoas muscle becomes populated with greater numbers of Type 2 fibers, identified by a larger size and greater force capacity, but capable of less endurance.

These Type 2 fibers support activity that is more related to sprinting, jumping and throwing, requiring quick reflexive actions—all activities necessary in stabilizing an erect, balanced posture. Interestingly enough, the opposite trend is noted in the small stabilizing multifidus muscles, where assumption of bipedal stance results in less demand for quick reflexive movement and the need for longer endurance support in these muscles, and, therefore, a population switch from Type 2 to Type 1 fibers.

One physiological action of the human psoas muscle is to flex the thigh, producing the high, powerful kicks seen in Can-Can dancers and football place-kickers. The other primary function is its role as the very powerful stabilizer of the pelvic girdle and lumbar vertebral segments—especially during walking, when the weight is momentarily supported on one leg or the other during transitional movements. The psoas muscle is also the muscle that comes under strain when we are tilted slightly forward while adjusting the weight of a heavy backpack.

As you might expect, it is a muscle of which we are almost completely unaware, working in the background as one of the major global stabilizers of our lower spine. If the knee is one of the "unsung heroes" in the discussion of joint anatomy, then the psoas muscle must certainly qualify for an equal award in the discussion of stabilization

Athletes who fail to stretch the psoas can experience deterioration in aerobic performance

of postural integrity. (The closest most of us have ever come to a psoas muscle, are the occasions of gastronomical delight marked by a filet mignon or tenderloin roast, benefited by the presence of a fine wine.)

It is the action of this very important muscle, however, that maintains the pelvic girdle in a level plane to support the foundation of posture. When performing optimally, the psoas muscle supports the curvature in the lower back, stabilizing the work of the lumbar vertebrae and exerting an upright tug on the front brim of the pelvis—much like a pair of internal suspenders keeping the pelvis centered under the weight of the overlying torso.

Because of our inattention to posture, most of us experience underperformance of the psoas muscle. On the other hand, athletic individuals who fail to take the time to stretch to overcome the effects of exercise, can often experience grief with strain patterns of the psoas muscle as it becomes shortened and overly tight.

In addition to development of postural aberrations with a tendency to tilt forward, these inattentive athletes will often feel tension between the shoulder blades, as well as burning sensations on the front of the thighs—especially during long walks or runs, or after prolonged periods of sitting. These same athletes may also experience deterioration in their aerobic performance as the tightened psoas has the ability to collapse the rib cage forward, inhibiting respiratory movement. Not uncommonly, if athletic trainers are unfamiliar with the role of the psoas muscle in supporting the postural integrity of the pelvic girdle, the origin and resolution of these problems will remain elusive to athletes and trainers alike.

Why the Pelvis Is the Third Most Important Contributor to Balance

Applying "The 3rd Step to Perfect Posture" involves becoming aware of the subtle, muscular control involved in keeping the pelvis tipped upward and maintaining the support of the pelvic girdle under the torso. The slight movements of the pelvic girdle in positioning itself under the weight of the torso are similar to the dynamic movements we have previously learned about in the movement of foot, ankle and knee.

Unlike the knee, foot, or ankle structural complexes in which the relatively large range of motion is easily appreciated, the movements of the pelvic girdle are far more delicate. To be kinaesthetically appreciated, they require greater focus on the subtle changes in muscular tension.

By keeping our mind's eye in the center of our pelvis during the application exercises, we can appreciate these small but powerful movements, the influence of the energy centers long recognized by Eastern mystics in their understanding of the functional integrity of the pelvis, and the contribution of the pelvis to our postural foundation.

Application Exercises

Stand with one leg on a thick book on the floor, while the opposite leg swings free alongside. Gently swing this leg back and forth at the hip joint, focusing on the psoas muscle attaching at its insertion point on the inner aspect of the upper thigh. Try and relax the big muscles at the front of the thigh, making the psoas do all the work.

Recognize the functional work of the psoas by forcibly pushing the lower stomach out while simultaneously attempting to lift the brim of the front of the pelvis against the strength of the pushing stomach wall. You will feel the tension in the psoas muscle at the lower end of the pelvis on the inside of the thigh where the psoas tendon passes through the groin and attaches to the upper inner thigh.

Imagine a carpenter's level running across the top of your pelvic girdle. Strive to keep the bubble in the middle, both while standing in one place and during movement.

Imagine the pelvic girdle as a floating basin resting on the pivot represented by the ball of your hip joints.

Imagine a billiard ball rolling around on the bottom of your pelvic basin. Move about, keeping the pelvic girdle basin as stable as possible and the billiard ball stationary at the bottom of the basin, not see-sawing back and forth while walking.

Reading Notes:

The 4th Secret: Keep Your Tailbone Tucked in

18

Many people present to their physician or therapist with the complaint that their tailbone hurts. When asked by their attending therapist to point towards the area of pain, they will invariably place their hand on a relatively large area of their backside encompassing the lower lumbar area as well as the central buttocks.

Given the large anatomical discrepancy represented by most people's description of the tailbone, it is probably best to break it down to the two bony structures forming it, commonly known as the sacrum and coccyx.

The Sacrum Is the First and Foundational Bone of the Spinal Column

The sacrum is a large, solid-appearing bone, shaped like an inverted pyramid. It forms the base of the spinal column, wedging into the back of the pelvic girdle much like a large boat snuggling into a V-shaped berth. At the very tip of the sacrum is the coccyx. This vestigial tail serves as an insertion point for many of the pelvic floor muscles that form a diaphragm, which supports the lower abdominal organs. The coccyx, representing the wiggly back-end of a goose, even in humans has a mobile joint where it connects to the end of the sacrum. It really has very little function at this stage in our evolution, other than to seemingly get in the way at the most inopportune times (ice skating, for example), resulting in contusion and injury, recognized in clinical practice as *coccygodynia*.

The mystical origins of the sacrum relate to our primordial "gut instincts"

The sacrum is situated at the very bottom of the spinal column, sometimes referred to as the *small of the back,* beginning at the top of the inter-gluteal cleft (less flatteringly known as the *butt crack).* The sacrum then curves gently downward and forward until it ends in a broad point articulating with the coccyx, a small bone about the size of your thumbnail.

Why the Sacrum Is Considered a Holy and Consecrated Bone

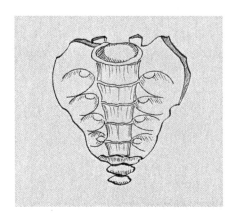

Os Sacrum, the Latin word describing this anatomical structure, translates as *holy* or *consecrated,* a derivation whose exact origin appears to have been lost to historical scholars. Many explanations have been put forth to support its origin. Rationalizations have ranged from its physical proximity to the sacred organs of procreation, to archaeological evidence pointing to its use as a vessel and shallow dish to hold sacrificial offerings. Some ancient civilizations believed that new life reassembled about the sacrum in the After-World, the sacrum being the last of the body to decay because of its large size. Surprisingly enough, many diverse cultures have independently attributed metaphysical qualities to the sacrum, many dating to times not recorded in written history.

Perhaps some of its mystical origins relate to the physiological significance referred to earlier, with its intimate physical relationship to the "second brain". The last of the spinal nerves, the four sacral nerves, flow outward through the foraminal openings in the sacrum, to contribute a significant component to the pelvic ganglion complex comprising the "second brain", responsible for autonomic abdominal organ function and the primordial *gut instincts* that we give credence to in our daily decision making.

In Traditional Chinese medicine (TCM), the sacrum is home to the beginning and most influential points of the Governing Vessel (Du Mai). Another "extraordinary meridian", the Du Mai is the most Yang of the meridians carrying Qi and the main vessel supplying Qi to the nervous system branching out from the spinal cord. The Governing Vessel is responsible for command, control and regulation of Qi in the remaining six subservient Yang channels. Interestingly enough, symptoms relating to dysfunction of the Du Mai meridian are reflected in stiff and painful spasms affecting the back and neck, made worse with movement and improved with rest.

In Taoist meditation practices, the energy of the Governing Vessel meridian comes alive with breathing techniques created to facilitate flow of Qi energy that starts from the tip of the coccyx and arises through the spinal column to the internal recesses of the brain where it nourishes the spiritual inner soul (Shen) along the Journey to Enlightenment.

In ancient Indian Tantric philosophy, at the very tip of the sacrum and coccyx, resting in the soft tissue of the pelvic floor called the *perineum*, is the home of the first Chakra, called by the Sanskrit name *Muladhara*. Muladhara is the root Chakra and the resting place of *Kundalini*, a serpent goddess whose energy force can be raised through ancient and esoteric meditation practices, resulting in a connection of all other chakras and an awakening of the rising psychic energy.

171

How the Human Sacrum has Evolved Differently from All Other Animals on Earth

The exact position of the sacrum is critical to the position of the rest of the spine

The sacrum has skeletally evolved in humans to show special adaptations in supporting the weight of erect man. Although wider and flatter in women, reflecting gender differences relating to its role in childbirth, the sacrum in both human sexes has more bony segments than other primates and possesses a wider, angulated base designed to support the increased axial load of upright ambulation.

Divided into five separate sacral vertebrae at birth, these vertebral segments will fuse together before adulthood, with involution of the intervertebral cartilaginous joints along the intervening discs, at which time after fusion, their separation in adulthood can only be detected by thin, vestigial lines noted on the front aspect of the sacrum.

The sacrum, thereafter, becomes the largest vertebral body upon which the foundation of the remaining spine, composed of 24 articulating vertebrae, must rest as it begins its ascension. The exact position and attitude of the sacrum, therefore, is critical to the eventual position of the rest of the spinal column. A slight change in sacral positioning becomes magnified in the curvature of the spinal segments positioned above it, to achieve a balanced, upright stance. This brings home the very truth noted earlier: *It is not possible to build a straight house on a crooked foundation.*

How a Baby's Spine Grows from a Fetal Position into a Perfect -Postured Spine in One Year

The development of the eventual curvatures noted in the human spine occur as an adaptation of the necessary bioengineering demands of supporting weight in an erect position.

During development in the womb, the spine develops in a single curvature, as identifyied in the developmental pictures of the fetus. Adoption of this curled-up position in adult life is still referred to as the *fetal position*. Within the first year of life, we develop all the four eventual curvatures of the spine, each anatomically identified as a *lordosis* if the curve has its convexity to the front, or *kyphosis* if the convexity faces backwards.

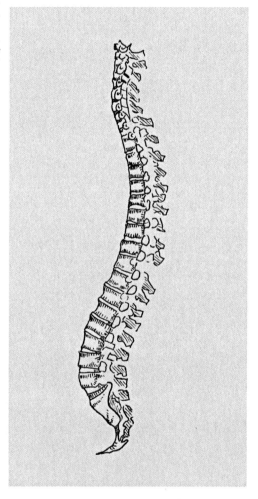

The first curvature developed is the cervical lordosis. This forward neck curvature is formed as the tottering infant balances its seemingly oversized head, eventually developing the strength to hold up the most massive brain developed in evolution. The second spinal curvature, called the lumbar lordosis, develops in the lower back. Again, it is a gentle forward curvature necessarily created to permit, first, sitting and, later, walking. Each of these forward curves will be balanced by a counterbalancing backward curve, already present from the single curve developed in the womb. The lower one, represented by the sacrum, creates the base for the lumbar lordosis. The thoracic curve creates a supporting backward-facing curve (kyphosis) running up to the junction where the neck starts.

In visualizing these four curves—two curving backwards in the sacrum and thoracic spine and two bending forward in the lumbar and cervical spine—we can see that they can be exaggerated or flattened. From a bioengineering stress standpoint, the flatter the curves, the less stress is placed on the ligaments as well as the musculature necessary in controlling upright stature. Accordingly, we should strive to institute whatever measures we can to flatten the curvatures and reduce the energy necessary to maintain erect stance.

How the Position of the Sacrum Controls the Entire Position of the Spine

The easiest way to do this is to control the *levelness* of the sacral platform. The anatomical range of motion of the sacrum is essentially a tipping motion, forward and back, with the pivotal point being the front lip of the top of the sacral platform, an anatomical movement referred to as *nutation* and *counternutation*.

> For ideal posture, our efforts should be directed at "tucking-in our tailbone"

There is a natural tendency in unconditioned individuals for the sacrum to tilt forward, which immediately sets up a platform necessitating excessive curvatures of the spine positioned above it. Therapists treating back pain will report this as an exaggerated lordosis, a condition often associated with chronic back pain and premature degenerative spondylosis representing a wearing out of the intervertebral discs between the vertebral bodies because of the added stress factors imposed on the spinal column.

Positioning of the sacrum, therefore, becomes critical in determining the eventual posture of the spinal column. For ideal postural positioning of the spine, our efforts should be directed at leveling the sacral platform, essentially *tucking our tailbone in* (picture a naughty pup with its tail between its legs).

Much like the directive of keeping the brim of the pelvis tipped up, the effect of tucking in the tailbone is, as well, a subtle kinesthetic experience—one requiring more conscious than physical effort. The first realization is that movement of the sacrum and coccyx is accomplished by a tightening of the pelvic floor musculature, which attaches to the sacrum and coccyx, much like a drum skin attaches to the surrounding rim.

To appreciate the movement of the sacrum, it is probably best to put the sacrum through its full range of motion of *nutation* and *counter-nutation*. By pushing the lower stomach out, you can feel the sacrum rocking forward with the tail-end coccyx sticking out backwards. Moving the sacrum in the opposite direction results in the top of the sacrum rocking backward and the tip of the tailbone following a forward curvilinear path, pointed at the ground.

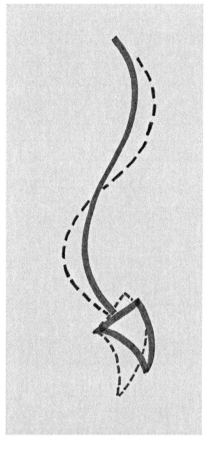

The most forward we can bring the coccyx in this curvilinear path would be demonstrated by a forceful contraction of the pelvic floor muscles, a sensation most of us have experienced when, after a long car ride and an extra-large coffee with high-fiber muffin, we hurriedly rush to the nearest bathroom.

Fortunately, it is unnecessary to bring that much force into play for correct positioning of the sacrum. What is necessary, however, is to gain an appreciation of the amount of control that we have in sacral movement using the muscles of the pelvic floor that constitute the pelvic diaphragm.

With the following application exercises, we will gain a significant appreciation of postural foundation as we learn control and implement "The 4th Secret of Perfect Posture".

Application Exercises

Re-live evolution in the fetal development of the four spinal curves. Start by putting your hands on your knees, bending forward to feel the curvatures developing in your lower and upper back and, finally, into your neck as your chin comes to rest against your chest. Now, slowly straighten your legs, letting your body drape itself backwards, feeling first the development of the forward curve of the lumbar lordosis and, lastly, the cervical lordosis as the head rests back, suspended by the muscles in the front of the neck.

Standing with your back against a wall, push the small of your back towards the wall in your best efforts to produce flattening of the lumbar lordosis.

Standing with your feet at shoulder width, imagine your tailbone pointing to the floor like a penlight in a darkened room. Using control of the pelvic floor muscles, imagine slowly drawing figure 8s on the floor between your legs, first in one direction and then the other. Appreciate the sizable range of motion that you are able to create in sacral movement.

While walking and standing, make an appreciable effort to keep the tailbone tucked in. This will flatten the lumbar lordosis and limit the excursion of the spinal curves above it, resulting in the least expended energy in maintenance of upright posture.

The 5th Secret: Let Your Chest Rise to the Sky

19

N o other anatomical structure of the human body—other than, perhaps, facial expression—is more indicative of the spirit of an individual than the carriage of their shoulders.

The recognizable shoulder posture of a person with confidence and energy is stark contrast to the position of obvious deference in a defeated individual, drooping forward, hunched, as if trying to slip through the imagined radar of intense, critical examination.

This posture of subservience is an inherited, evolutionary behavior and is seen not only in primates but also in other lower classes of the animal kingdom. Although it may have some survival value in the lower animal kingdom in the avoidance of aggression from superior peers, for reasons that have been clearly outlined it is neither necessary nor desirable in modern society. Efforts should be continuously made to correct any tendency towards assumption of this aberrant posture.

What Do Military Parades, Poets and Sculpturors have in Common?

Not surprisingly, therefore, shoulder girdle posture is the key position addressed in military parades. The appearance and perfection of shoulder alignment has been important throughout the ages in showcasing the aesthetic appreciation of fashion, in clothing as well as in serving as a gallery of display for some of the most priceless objects of art ever designed. The alluring curves formed by the shoulders and neck easily catch our eye and have for centuries fascinated artists, sculptors, poets and fashion designers alike, providing an exquisite venue for their artistry.

> Clavicles and scapulae together form a bioengineering feat made even more remarkable when heavy loads are added to the job

When we speak about the shoulder girdle, we are talking about two, distinct structures, structurally connected and moving in concert. The first structure, the rib cage, describes the 12 ribs, which articulate both in the front with a large triangular bone called the *sternum* or breastbone, and at the back with the 12 thoracic vertebrae forming the dorsal spinal column. Forming a protective enclosure that guards the lungs, heart and great vessels from blunt injury, the rib cage is relatively fixed but has a definitive range of motion describing its expansion and retraction with respiratory movement.

The second structure comprising the shoulder girdle includes the shoulder blades or *scapulae*, and collarbones or *clavicles*. The clavicles form joints at each of their ends, articulating with the top of the breastbone and, at the other end, toward the shoulder, with the scapulae.

As seen from above, the combination of scapulae and clavicles takes on the appearance of a squished, elliptical hoop. This "squished hoop" provides all the attachment points for the muscles forming the shoulder girdle, which, as a unit, will drape over the underlying rib cage like the midnight-black cape of Zorro.

The shoulder girdle, sitting above the rib cage, moves over the rib cage as if suspended on an air cushion—up and down as we shrug, and forward and back when we either stand at attention or slump forward in defeat.

The movement of the rib cage itself is quite straightforward and illustrates the movement defined by the natural rhythm of inhalation and expiration. With inhalation, the ribs lift upward and outward, while at the same time the muscular diaphragm, which forms a drum encasing the bottom end of the rib cage, pushes downward and outward.

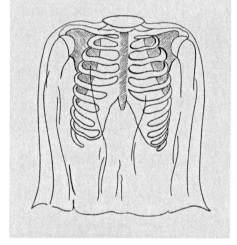

Letting our air out, or expiration, is a passive, relaxed response whereupon the air in the lungs gently pushes out as we relax the musculature, the natural elasticity of the interconnecting muscles and ligaments between the ribs pulling the walls of the rib cage back to center.

Clavicles and scapulae together form a complex counterbalancing configuration, permitting independent, 360°, three-dimensional movement of the arms. That this bioengineering feat is possible at all is remarkable; however, greater still, the human shoulder and arm can also accomplish this range of motion while at the same time loaded with heavy weights and forces.

This is only possible because of the complicated muscular organization controlling the movement of the scapulae bones, large triangular cancellous bones gliding on the back of the rib cage like inverted plates and functioning as counter-weights that allow the arms to be lifted effortlessly in the multi-dimensional movement we enjoy.

The shoulder blades are tethered by large, muscular groups, which attach to the spine and the shoulder on each side, as well as being suspended from above and below. This complete circumferential muscular attachment allows the scapulae to move upwards and downwards, outward and inward, and even rotate as it produces its complicated counterweight activity to support arm movement and contribute to the strength of the shoulder.

So, now that we can appreciate the purpose of the shoulder girdle, what is the best postural position we can adopt to ensure maximal ergonomic function?

How Tension in the Shoulders Throws Off Posture and Creates the Dreaded "Sniff Position"

The first consideration is that the shoulder must work in a tension-free environment for maximum efficiency. In most of us, the first symptom of stress will be a tightening of the trapezius muscles at the back of the shoulder girdle and neck, where the upper-dorsal 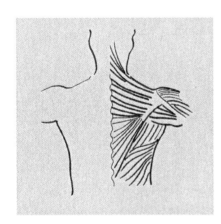 vertebral column makes its junctional transition into the neck. This is the tense muscle at the top of the shoulders that feels so good when massaged, providing that intense sensation of relaxation.

This anatomical area called the *thoracocervical junction* is a key stress area in most of us, serving almost like a "tension barometer". In the worst-case scenario, the tension can be so great, we feel like our shoulders are being pulled up to our ears like earmuffs on a cold day. Just being aware of this tendency is often enough of a reminder to allow us to consciously relax our trapezius muscles draping across the top of our shoulders, letting the scapulae drop back down into the functional position they belong.

Failure to allow the scapulae to operate in this functional position results in a forward-bowed position of the shoulder girdle throwing the whole balance of posture forward. This results in the neck extending forward in the "sniff position", so-called because of the appearance of a person trying to locate the source of a bad odor. Almost always, these people will have chronic tension patterns in the muscles of the upper back and neck, often associated with chronic muscular-contraction headaches developing towards the later part of the day. These symptoms will most always relate to the extra muscular work of holding the head in this aberrant pose.

The headache pattern associated with this pose is often described as an ache that starts at the back of the head and neck and, over-time, creeps over the top of the head, into the forehead, ultimately creating a tightening sensation that feels like wearing a hat that is three sizes too small.

This forward rolling position of the shoulders also results in a collapse of the front of the rib cage, with restriction of inspiratory movement, resulting in a decrease in lung tidal volume. Reduced capacity for oxygenation and exhalation of waste carbon dioxide may likely be contributary factors responsible for the increased fatigue levels often experienced.

> Slouching results in a collapse of the rib cage, reducing oxygenation and increasing fatigue

The Key to Correct Shoulder-Girdle Posture Is Relaxation

Relaxation of the scapular muscles and avoidance of rigidity in the shoulder girdle, allows the scapulae to drop down and drift towards the midline, placing them into the ideal functional position. One should keep the feeling that the shoulder girdle is floating over the rib cage, separated like a hydrofoil boat over water.

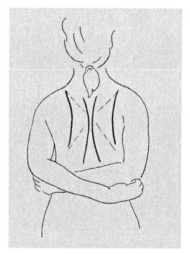

There is a tendency to want to achieve this by tugging the shoulder blades together at the back to create an "at attention" pose. This tendency should be avoided as it encourages tension in the shoulder girdle interfering with the freedom of scapular movement. It is enough to merely relax the muscles of the shoulder girdle. This in itself will permit the full range of motion in its inherent design.

Correct positioning of the rib cage provides the rest of the formula for the ideal shoulder girdle posture. Thinking of the endpoint of the rib cage at full inspiration gives us the best kinesthetic appreciation of ideal positioning. The lower ribs should be gently pushed forward and the upper ribs should be lifted towards the sky. If you test this movement by repeatedly inhaling and exhaling, performing these two instructions of pushing the lower ribs forward and lifting the upper ribs up, you can feel that the fulcrum upon which the rib cage rocks is the junction where the upper lumbar vertebrae meet the lower thoracic vertebrae, a key anatomical point called the *thoracolumbar junction*.

Keeping this position without allowing the rib cage to collapse on itself, while maintaining a relaxed but ready, supporting shoulder-girdle musculature is the correct postural position for maximum ergonomic function. Finding that balance without the tension is key to "The 5th Secret of Perfect Posture".

Application Exercises

Position your rib cage and shoulder girdle in the ideal position. Practice the ancient meditative breathing rhythm, allowing the lungs to fill and the rib cage to expand by consciously pushing the diaphragm downward towards the pelvic floor. Feel the lower ribs push out and the upper ribs lift as the lungs fill to their full capacity.

Holding the ideal shoulder girdle posture, place your arms out in front of your body and begin making small concentric circles, enlarging them very gradually. Do this in both a clockwise and counter-clockwise direction, appreciating the counterbalancing circular movement of the scapulae gliding across the back of the rib cage.

With your arms down by your sides, very slowly roll your shoulders in a circular movement forward and then backwards, appreciating the freedom of the full range of motion of the shoulder girdle draped over the rib cage.

To appreciate the absence of tension in the ideal shoulder girdle posture, imagine helium balloons tucked underneath the diaphragm, floating the rib cage and the shoulder girdle upwards.

Reading Notes:

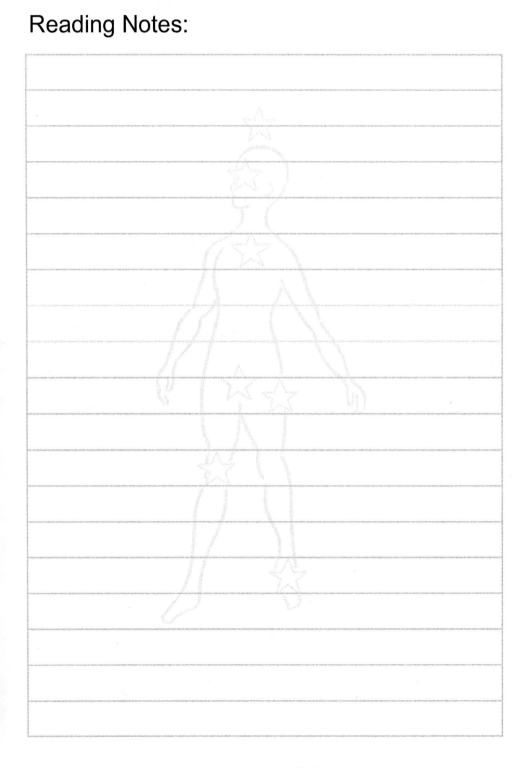

The 6th Secret: Keep Your Eyes on the Horizon

T he eyes have always held a particular fascination in human history and even today are thought by many to be "windows to the soul". Most certainly, they have played a critical role in social evolution, with permission of eye contact between individuals indicative of peer status, not only in humans, but also in lower members of the animal kingdom.

Through the ages, considerable time and effort have been spent embellishing the eyes for personal adornment. Given their social importance, it is not unreasonable that we ascribe various emotions to the eyes' appearance during human interaction: glaring, alluring, seducing, piercing, or compassionate, to name a few. When asked what the specific distinction in the different eye appearances is, most of us would be at a loss to explain the emotional input that brings us to our answer, our reaction being more *"gut"* than observational. Clearly, eye communication is far more complex than appears at first glance (no pun intended).

The Amazing Evolution of Human Vision

In humans, the eyes are set deeply in cone-shaped orbital sockets, facing forward and slightly outward, creating an overlap of visual fields that permit binocular vision and depth of perception. Our small nose accentuates this visual-field overlap, allowing us to see downwardly in our peripheral vision as well.

In addition to their function as the organs of sight, the eyeballs are also neurologically connected to the pituitary gland deep within the brain. Both light and visual stimulation influence hormonal levels in our body. Some of these hormones may be produced immediately, based on the visual picture in front of us. Other hormone levels are more gradually changed, based on circadian or seasonal rhythms.

The human evolutionary development of the head situated on top of the spine, with the ability to rotate to each side as well as up and down, was a significant breakthrough that gave ancient man the capability of seeing greater distances over the horizon. This imparted significant survival improvements over man's predecessors, both in the ability to search for food as well as vigilance for possible enemies.

By far, vision plays the most critical role in postural balance

This new placement of the head on top of the spine, although significantly beneficial for vision, created new problems in postural design. With the head now perched higher on the skeleton, bioengineering problems are created secondary to the high center of gravity relative to the rest of the body. There becomes less room for error, with any deviations from optimal head alignment creating significant impact on the entire body's postural balance.

Why the Eyes Are the Most Important Contributor to Balance

This ability to maintain postural balance is affected by even slight changes in head position, with laboratory studies showing minor flexion or extension of the head from normal upright position significantly affecting the body's ability to maintain normal postural balance. The role of our eyes provides critical assistance in postural balance to overcome this factor. Visually fixating on the horizon provides us with the necessary criteria for *optical righting*, an innate reflex inherited phyllogenetically from the lower animal kingdom.

For ideal postural balance, it is best, therefore, to have the head in neutral balance with the eyes fixed on the horizon, a point of fact not lost on any dancer or figure skater in the process of performing the complex turns and spins in the fundamental choreography of the art form.

To support the visual contribution to balance, nature has also provided an extraordinarily rich number of proprioceptive sensory nerve endings in our neck region, both in the muscles as well as in the joints, providing a constant feedback loop to the brain, assisting in movement control and alignment.

By far, however, vision plays the most critical part in postural balance, outweighing even the vestibular contribution of the inner ear. The contribution of vision to balance can easily be demonstrated by the difference in ease of standing on one leg, with or without our eyes closed.

How the Tongue Helps Free Neck Movement

One other point not commonly discussed regarding head position and contribution to postural balance, is that neutral plane alignment and balance of the head on the cervical spine requires relaxation of the major muscles controlling jaw movement. Marked tension in the strong biting masseter and temporalis muscles at the top of the jaw and temple where the mandible joins the skull, and even the muscles controlling the tongue, will restrict the ability of the head to pivot freely on the top of the spine. For this reason, dancers and skaters are always encouraged by coaches to be aware of this fact and make conscious effort to relax the muscles around the jaw and mouth during performances.

The 7 Secrets of Perfect Posture

"The 6th Secret of Perfect Posture" is recognizing the pivotal role of postural foundation and balance played by fixing our visionary 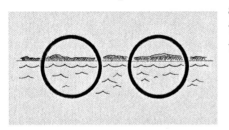 axis on the horizon, keeping the head in neutral balance while maintaining relaxation of the very important facial and jaw muscles.

Application Exercises

To kinaesthetically feel the neutral balance of ideal head position over the cervical spine, produced by relaxation of the involved muscles, practice the following exercise. With your eyes closed, touch the tip of your tongue gently against the roof of your mouth, just behind your front teeth, with the teeth slightly held apart. Hold this position for a few seconds, with your focus following the relaxation pattern as it settles into the muscles controlling the jaw and face. In this position, the muscles controlling the jaw and face must automatically relax, taking out any existing tension in the muscles.

For perfect positioning of the eyes on the horizon, imagine floating in an upright position in a pool of water, where the eyeballs are half in and half out of the water. This produces a visual picture like the ones we have seen in National Geographic nature programs, where one half of the picture is under the water, and the other half is looking above the water. Feel how the chin is slightly tucked without creating any tension in the back of the neck.

For effortless rotation of the head on the cervical spine, a good visual exercise is to imagine the head to be a helium-filled balloon tugging gently upward on the top of the spine. From this vantage point, it is effortless for the head to rotate on the spine.

Reading Notes:

The 7th Secret: Feel the Lift from Within

The previous six secrets have been specific, kinesthetic clues to body positioning to help us find the correct postural alignment for foundation integrity. The last and "7th Secret of Perfect Posture" is a command to our inner physiology, a call to conscious vigilance bringing about a sense of attention and alertness.

In an earlier section, we discussed the contribution to posture of Chong Mai, the Traditional Chinese Medicine (TCM) "extraordinary meridian" responsible for maintenance of postural alignment and the internal vertical axis of the body. We learned that the Chong Mai meridian stems from the Earth below, flowing into the base of the inner foot and coursing up the insides of our legs into the spinal canal, progressing upward into the inner recesses of the brain.

We also recall that the strength and vitality of this meridian is a hereditary force, shared and absorbed from the communal life force that surrounds us. This life energy manifested in the body is the result of the many unseen life functions maintained by our autonomic nervous system (ANS), keeping our hearts beating, maintaining effortless breathing, controlling our body's temperature and absorbing and converting the nutrients we eat into the energy we require continuously to rejuvenate our living cells.

Tapping into the Ancient Postural Energy Streams

The English translation of Chong Mai into *thoroughfare* or *heavenly cord*, alludes to an axis of energy that courses through us like an *artery of vitality*, connecting us not only to the Earth below but suspending us from the Heavens above, making available to us the energy of both. The ancient Chinese Masters believed that it was possible for us to tap into this energy, working in concert with it to enhance our own life force. It was for this purpose that the exercise routines of Taijiquan and Qigong were developed in the earliest times of human civilization.

The breathing exercises and physical movements were designed to assist the individual in recognizing this constant flow of energy that we absorb from the Earth below, filling our body with uplifting energy, with the nourishment of each living cell. The air that we breathe is as important as the food that we eat, and management of breathing through conscious effort and diaphragmatic control remains paramount in both athletic and meditative practices for maximum performance and affect.

Lengthening our outward breathing changes our physiological state and calms the mind

Recognizing that no practice continues for thousands of years without some remedial value, what particular knowledge is in this health practice that has been preserved and passed down that can be useful to us in maintenance of healthy posture?

Breathing patterns are greatly influenced by one's internal, psychological state; conversely, changing breathing patterns can alter our existing psychological state.

How Breathing Can Change Our Inner Physiology

During relaxed inhalation, we should feel the diaphragm gently pushing downward and outward, allowing the lungs within to expand. This downward and outward pushing sensation of the diaphragm can be felt not only within the respiratory diaphragm, but the pelvic floor as well, which also functions like a diaphragm gently pushing downward at the same time.

We can feel the efforts of these two diaphragmatic support structures working in concert to provide strength, as evidenced by the tension we would feel in both during the efforts of pushing against a solid wall. Failure of the integrity of this pelvic floor diaphragm is a major cause of urinary incontinence, a significant problem for many women, especially following childbirth.

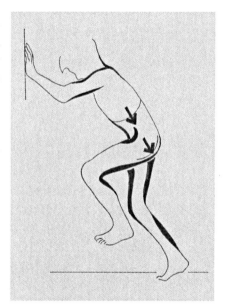

Exhalation under conditions other than during exertion results from relaxation of these muscles and contraction of the diaphragm, compressing the lungs and gently pushing the air out through the exiting passages.

Many reproducible laboratory studies have demonstrated that lengthening the expiration phase of the respiratory cycle results in changes in our physiological state, resulting in a calming effect upon the mind, whereas shortening the exhalation reflects urgency to our physiological state with equally predictable results.

Awareness of these physiological effects associated with breathing patterns allows us to control the physical and emotional tension in our body, using breathing techniques to influence our physiological and psychological states. Dependent on our needs, the outcome states may either be calming *or* invigorating, but personal empowerment is attained in the knowledge that we *can* exercise this control and need not be a victim of our own internal states.

Although there may be situations whereby there is a need to intensify and invigorate energy states, such as prior to an athletic event, more often it is necessary to move our physiology in the opposite direction, restraining overreaction and inducing a more steady state that permits our bodies to take adequate time to assess a situation before reacting.

> **It is the acknowledgment of personal empowerment and control over our physiological state that we want to develop**

Everything in Moderation Including Moderation

This is the arena of Chong Mai: the role of the autonomic nervous system (ANS) is that of the moderator, finding the equilibrium in life that represents neither too much nor too little. Finding middle ground is a challenge that most of us struggle with in one aspect of our life or another. If only our lives could consistently reflect that balance: *Everything in moderation, including moderation.* There is little in life so damaging that, if practiced in moderation, it will cause much harm.

It is the acknowledgment of personal empowerment and control over our physiological state that we want to develop. The entrainment of these biofeedback skills is the enigma of Chong Mai discovered early in civilization by intuitive masters. Whereas knowledge of these practices in ancient civilizations was restricted to select protégés, passed down secretly from generation to generation, today the body of knowledge regarding our ability to change our inner state is growing in leaps and bounds as scientists unravel the mystery of the neurophysiology of the human body.

To put this knowledge to use, however, the practices must involve taking the time to listen to our body, becoming intuitive to our needs and looking within for change rather than without. It is an acknowledgment of connectedness to the Earth and to the Heavens—-and being aware of the energy emanating from both.

All of us at some time or another have made this connection—even if only momentarily. In this moment, Chong Mai comes alive.

In this frozen moment of time, there is a very real kinesthetic appreciation, a springing of muscle and tendon, a lightness to our step with a feeling of rejuvenation, and a recognition of the life force that infuses us. Every cell of our body appears to be a sensory antenna to the environment around us, contributing individually and collectively to the interaction of life surrounding us.

For this moment, there is an appreciation of the flow of energy connecting us with Heaven and Earth, filling our body with uplifting energy and the confidence to hold the ground on which we stand.

The difference between the Great Masters and us is that they have strung more of these moments together than we have. While it may be true that today we are probably more preoccupied than we have ever been in the history of civilization, it is equally important to recognize that if we are too busy to take the time to look after our own needs, we are probably just ...

"Too Busy!"

We owe a responsibility to ourselves and the care of our bodies. Becoming aware of the energy that surrounds us and its interaction with our own energy system is the first step, an empowering action that will enhance our life many times over as we begin the journey that marks the rest of our life.

Practice the exercises of the "7th Secret to Perfect Posture" and "Feel the Lift From Within."

Application Exercises

Stand barefoot in the grass and close your eyes. Feel the solidness of the Earth and the texture of the ground beneath your feet. Feel the tingling of your scalp from the movement of the surrounding air. Let your senses appreciate the energy that surrounds and infuses you. In your mind's eye, see yourself as an extension of life's energy represented in the vast universe of the infinite time, space and energy that surrounds us.

Imagine a vertical line beginning on the floor between your feet, moving up through your legs into the center of your body, rising through the spinal column to the top of your head, suspending you from the sky above. Infuse this vertical axis with the power from the Earth pushing up through your legs, your elongated spine and your head suspended from above as the *Heavenly Cord* continues to the heavens.

Create an anatomical model in your mind, in which a helium channel is infused into the core of your weight-bearing skeleton, providing buoyancy and spring. Imagine, as well, disks of helium supporting the pelvic floor and chest diaphragm, and a small helium prayer cap over the skull—all providing that inner vertical lift of Chong Mai.

Awakening Chong Mai makes us feel taller, more vital and alert—a sensory preparedness that is constantly evident in nature around us. Imagine a sentinel prairie dog perched alertly on the top of his mound, peering over the horizon with watchful eyes; or an eagle perched on a nest, undistracted by her fussy brood, the attention of her entire being fixed, undivided, on the source of the family's next meal.

PART IV

THE **7** STEPS TO
PERFECT POSTURE

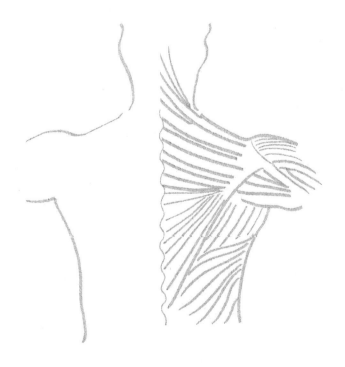

The 7 Steps to Perfect Posture

22

S
T
E
P
S

T he 7 steps to perfect posture may very likely be the easiest to understand of all the material presented thus far, but likely the most difficult to implement. This is not necessarily because of their complexity, but because, like all new things we try to implement in our lives, there is a certain inertia that has to be overcome in beginning the journey. However, as we all know, each journey only begins with the courage to take the first step.

We've made the commitment to come this far and, as noted earlier, the reasonable person will always entertain the possibility that a new approach may be helpful in resolving an old problem.

Give "The 7 Steps to Perfect Posture" a try! The worst-case scenario is that your chronic back pain and posture will remain unchanged; however, the odds are much greater that your efforts will be rewarded by all the promises of improved posture.

1. Do Your Homework

Many people will start a project, often with little background knowledge of the goals that they are attempting to achieve, hoping to "wing it" and pick up the knowledge along the way. Others, in fact, feel that this is the only way to begin a new project, inasmuch as any other approach stifles creativity and results in fewer options being explored.

Most would agree, however, that a review of the known information, establishing a firm base of knowledge, shortens the learning curve and gives the project a measurable time line, a plan that is far more likely to reduce the number of little frustrations that will surface along the way.

If you have read the material in this book, you likely have all the information required to implement the changes necessary to achieve perfect posture.

2. Be Gentle With Yourself

As any experienced therapist who has worked with patients in dealing with chronic back pain and postural problems knows, a dilemma that consistently comes up is the tendency for patients to overdo the exercise prescriptions given to them.

This is probably only a natural, human response. Having made the effort and the commitment to address a problem, the first resolution that we will probably make is that, if this is the route that we must take, then we'd best get at it!

> Resist the natural, human response to "overdo" the Seven Steps

Such an approach will result in predictable consequences. The previously unchallenged muscles will complain most vigorously if we overextend our initial efforts, resulting in an inflammatory flare-up with all the accompanying symptoms.

There is only one solution and that is to carefully follow the *10% rule*. Start at a level that you absolutely know will cause you no difficulties. Increase your program by no more than 10% every third work out, either in repetitions *or* effort—*but not both*!

"Rome was not built in a day!"

Having said that, I'm reminded of an impatient patient who retorted

"I know that *but...I wasn't foreman on that job!"*

3. You Can't Stretch Enough

Believe it or not, the problem with correcting postural foundation is not likely strength, but most probably our soft tissue malleability preventing the full range of motion of the affected weight-bearing axial skeletal joints. Most of us have plenty of strength and, in fact, too much strength in the muscles that we use all day long.

It is this imbalance between the muscles of our prime movers and the muscles that oppose their action that prevent most of us from assuming normal postural stance.

The classic example that applies to most of us is the imbalance between the strength of the muscles of our chest and the muscles between our shoulder blades, giving us the tendency to roll our shoulders forward. Another example is the tightness of the muscles in the back of our thighs preventing us from comfortably sitting in a 90° position on a flat surface with our legs extended out in front of us.

> Believe it or not, our problem isn't *strength* it's *stretch*!

A good rule of thumb is that we should spend at least 10 minutes *before* every exercise session and 10 minutes *after* every exercise session with a first-rate stretching program to ensure our muscles aren't *interfering* with our postural foundation.

4. Increase Your Core Power

Two things give us the strength to get through our day with minimal fatigue: the first is aerobic fitness and the second, our core strength.

Aerobic fitness defines the ability of our body to use oxygen efficiently in cellular metabolism. We achieve aerobic fitness by challenging our cardiac and respiratory systems to perform at the upper levels of their capability. These levels are dependent on our age and other parameters of our health status. Efforts at achieving these fitness levels can be accomplished with as little as 30 minutes participation in an aerobic exercise program each day. We should all be encouraged to work at maintenance of aerobic fitness providing there is no medical contraindication.

Core power defines the muscular strength responsible for postural stabilization of the axial skeletal system. There are a great number of exercise programs that promote core stability and no one system is likely superior to another. What is important, however, is that you find the exercise program challenging and entertaining enough to sustain interest in attendance, because discontinuation will result in a 10% loss of fitness within a two-week period.

The sooner we realize that success will depend on a lifetime commitment to maintenance of core strength, the easier it becomes.

The other thing to remember is:

A change is as good as a rest!

There are many different core stabilization programs out there, from swimming laps to Pilates and yoga. Mix it up and keep yourself interested and challenged!

5. Practice, Practice, Practice

As the New York cabbie told the tourist inquiring as to how to get to Carnegie Hall, "Practice! Practice! Practice!"

Kinesthetic learning is available to everyone willing to put in the effort

There are few things in life that come easily without repeated effort, and postural foundation is no exception.

There is a principle referred to in physical training, called *muscle memory*. This concept refers to the body's ability to remember its position relative to space and time.

A repeated, specific postural position returned to over time will result in each involved joint developing an awareness of the exact weight-bearing point within that specific joint. The muscles that control that joint will recognize the exact tension and strength required to maintain the joint in that position.

This kinesthetic learning experience is dependent on the amount of time spent on the task at hand but will consistently come about within given parameters of time to every person willing to put in the effort.

Unfortunately, there is little substitution for the New York cabbie's advice—we'll just have to put in the time!

6. Stand Your Ground

There comes a time in everyone's life when we have to take a stand, dig in our heels and accept that retreat is not an option. It is a recognition that there are some things in life that, unless we do them for ourselves, will remain undone.

Taking responsibility for maintaining perfect posture and, for that matter, our health in general can't be anyone else's responsibility; it must necessarily be our own. It is only too easy to delegate responsibility, whether it be to a physician for a prescription that will hopefully resolve our problem, or a therapist to give us a treatment that can be passively applied without any input on our part to effect the outcome.

In postural foundation at least, the result will only come about because of the efforts we commit ourselves to undertake. Regardless of the number and variety of postural foundation belts, postural seating supports or contoured pillows we trial, in the end, the best results will come from our own efforts to change our postural alignment.

The sooner we come to this conclusion, the sooner we can move in a direction of change. Someone once defined lunacy as doing the same things over and over again, with expectations of a different result. Personal empowerment and taking responsibility for the choices that we make is our best bet to ensure that we become the beneficial recipient of the promises of perfect posture.

7. Pay Attention

All of us, at one time or another, are surprised to find how much can happen around us, things that we can be completely oblivious to, having screened it from our conscious awareness. Whether it is because our mind is focused on the deliberation of a specific problem or we have unconsciously tuned out the *pitter-patter of life* surrounding us, the end result is that both time and the world have passed us by—and it has happened without any mindful decision on our part.

Certainly our inattention to posture falls into this category. In the beginning, we will probably find ourselves constantly needing reminders to trigger the kinesthetic clues we have covered in the maintenance of ideal posture, to achieve the goal of improving our postural alignment. Paying attention will seem like quite a chore at first but, with persistence, habitual patterns after a time will begin acting in our favor in the overall achievement of our established goals.

The advice to *pay attention* is good practice for life in general, for attention and commitment to details, especially when it comes to health, are critical in determining outcomes. Whereas under other circumstances in life, this benign neglect may not be injurious, this inattention may be very harmful—especially when it comes to ignoring habitual patterns that may impact negatively on our personal health.

"The great tragedy of life is that most people die with their music still in them."
Goethe

Most often, inattention to our life's details is a carelessness in establishing priorities, a reflection of the common tendency towards procrastination that affects many of us. Almost all of us will give our attention to those things that we find most pressing in our lives for that moment, putting out the fires likely to overwhelm us. Often, however, what we find most pressing may not in fact be the most important thing that we should be addressing. Perhaps our focus would be better directed to the cause of the fire rather than the noticeable flames.

There is a quote attributed to the German philosopher Goethe: "The great tragedy of life is that most people die with their music still in them." Making the effort to commit the necessary attention to our posture and health *by taking action now,* underlines our responsibility to ourselves. In taking this action, we have at least the satisfaction of knowing that we have done all that we can to alter the outcome.